AF526495

HUMAN ANATOMY AND PHYSIOLOGY, TEXT BOOK (BP101T)

Rajesh Kumar Mukherjee,
Dr. Dilip Kumar Roy.

First printing edition, 2024
Distribution rights to all territories (Worldwide rights)

9 789334 035186

ISBN 13: 978-93-340-3518-6

Copyright©2012 Rajesh Kumar Mukherjee
All rights reserved.

Dedication

This book is completely devoted to those individuals (Students) who continuously struggle to compete in this competitive world with truth by following the right path, don't try to harm others and try to live peacefully.

Most of the people during their challenging periods of my life are self-constrict themselves and we the authors of this book striving to surpass our limits and present our achievements in the form of this book to everyone who aspires to improve themselves and enhance their abilities and knowledge.

Regular expressions of gratitude or encouragement can significantly improve someone's life in a unique and elevated manner.

Thank You Everyone.

Content page

Topic	Page no.
Unit 1: Human Body (Cellular and tissue level of organization)	06 – 58
Unit 2: Integumentary system, skeleton system and joints	60 – 89
Unit 3: Blood fluids and lymphatic system	91 – 108
Unit 4: Peripheral nervous system and special sense organs	110 – 132
Unit 5: Cardiovascular System	134 – 158

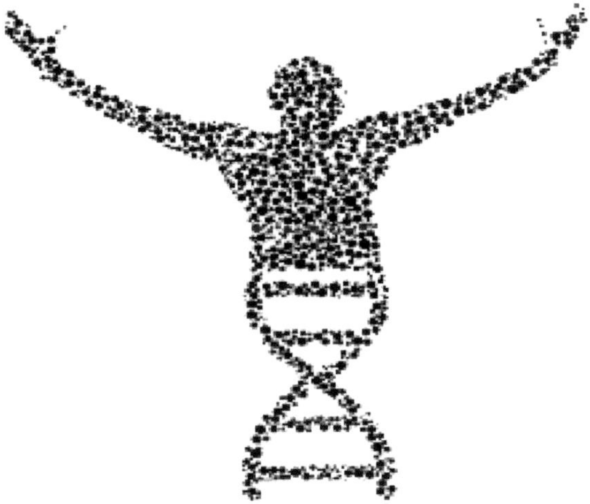

About the authors

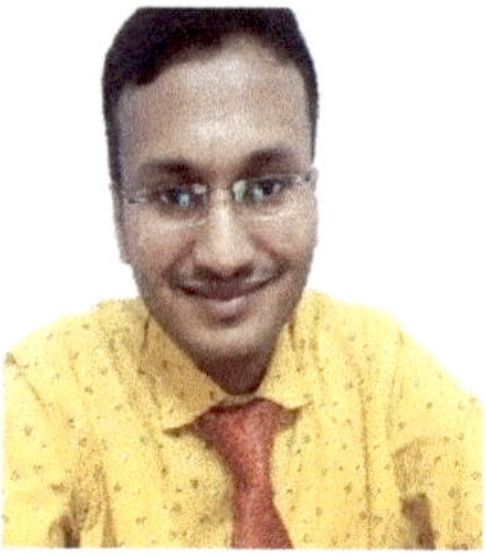

Mr. Rajesh Kumar Mukherjee, a Research Scholar (pursuing Ph.D. in Pharmacology from JIS University, Kolkata, West Bengal, India), has 3.10 years of industrial experience (R&D Analytical Development Laboratory and Pharmacovigilance) and 3.8 years of academic experience (currently working as an Assistant Professor in Brainware University, Department of Pharmaceutical Technology, Barasat, West Bengal, India). He has published 2 books, 2 patents, and a and a few research articles in reputed journals and secured lots of oral and poster presentation awards at the national and international levels.

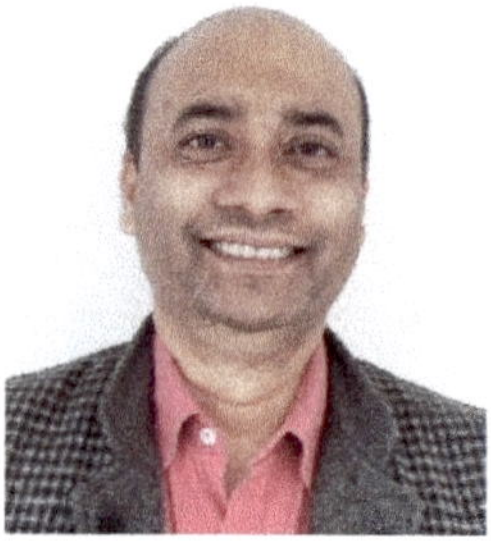

Dr. Dilip Kumar Roy, M. Pharm, Ph. D. from Jadavpur University, has renounced expertise for around 18 years in the Pharma and Biotech Industries (R&D) and 3+ years of academic experience (currently working as an Associate Professor at JIS University, Department of Pharmaceutical Technology, Kolkata, West Bengal, India). He has published more than 10+ review and research articles in reputed journals, 4+ books, and patents to his credit, secure awards in national and international levels, as well as guided a lot of Ph. D., M. Pharm, and B. Pharm students.

Unit 1.

Topic	Page no.
Chapter 1: Introduction to human body	06 – 12
1.1. Definition and scope of anatomy and physiology	12 – 14
1.2. Levels of structural organization in the human body	14 – 17
1.3. Basic life processes	17
1.4. Homeostasis	18 – 20
1.5. Basic anatomical terminology	20 – 22

Topic	Page no.
Chapter 2: Cellular level of organization	22 – 25
2.1. Structure and functions of cell	25 – 27
2.2. Transport across cell membrane	27 – 29
2.3. Cell division	29 – 31
2.4. Cell junctions	32 – 33
2.5. General principles of cell communication	33 – 34
2.6. Intracellular signaling pathway activation by extracellular signal molecule	35 – 37
2.7. Forms of intracellular signaling: (Contact-dependent, paracrine, synaptic, endocrine)	37 – 44

Topic	Page no.
Chapter 3: Tissue level of organization	45 – 51
3.1. Structure, location and functions of epithelial tissue	51 – 53
3.2. Structure, location and functions of muscular tissue	53 – 55
3.3. Structure, location and functions of nervous tissue	55 – 56
3.4. Structure, location and functions of connective tissue	56 – 57

Related questions from unit 1	58

Unit 1.

Chapter 1.
Introduction to human body

The human body is a vital complex system comprised of interconnected structures and organs that processes and collaborate to maintain life and balancing homeostasis throughout this entire living body, once it drastically affected and the pathological changes doesn't alter to normal at that last stage the affected miserable living system becomes slows downs to death, below are some key features and systems.

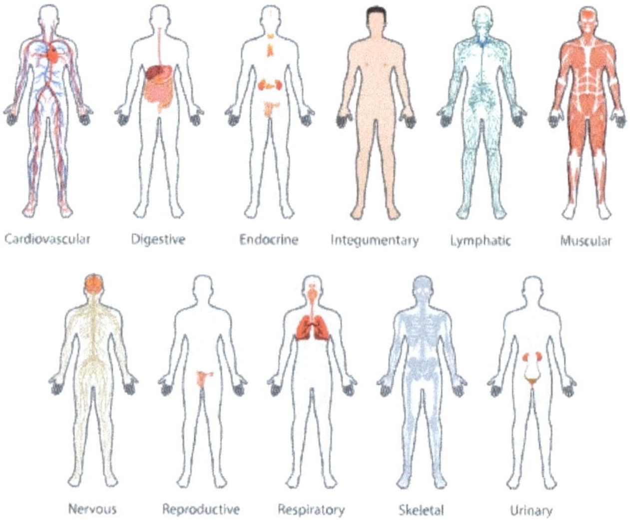

Fig. 1. Human body systems.

i. Skeletal system: The skeletal system is the anatomical structure that involves bones and connective tissues. It plays a role in the production of red blood cells, mineral accumulation, movement, and overall body function, and it provides structure, support, and protection.

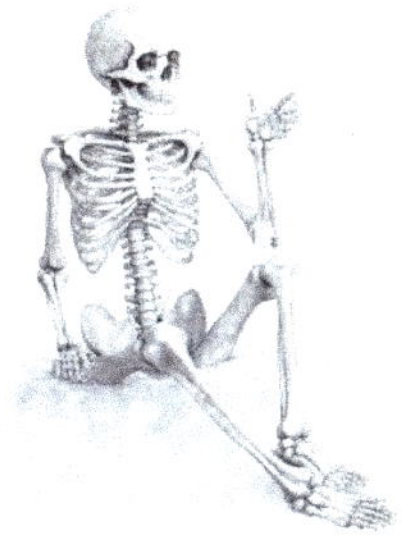

Fig. 2. Skeletal system.

a. Bone serves to maintain structural integrity, offer support, safeguard interior organs, and enable movement. (There are total 206 bones in human body)
b. Joints facilitate the movement and flexibility of the body. (There are total 350 joints in human body)
c. Cartilage: Offers both cushioning and structural support to joints. (There are total 3 cartilages in human body)

ii. Muscular system: The musculoskeletal system is composed of a multifaceted collection of muscles that facilitate movement, stability, and the maintenance of essential physiological functions by contracting and relaxing muscles. It is essential for both voluntary and involuntary internal movement.

a. Muscles: It facilitate movement by undergoing contraction and relaxation. (There are total 600 muscles in human body)
b. Tendons: Muscles facilitate the connection between
bones and muscles. (There are total 4000 tendons in human body)
c. Ligament: establish connections between bones. (There are total 900 ligaments in human body)

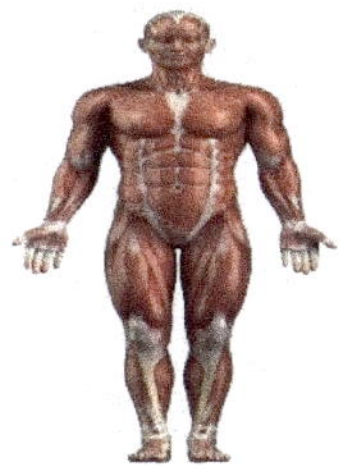

Fig. 3. Muscular system.

iii. Circulatory system: The cardiovascular system also referred to as the circulatory system, is responsible for the transportation of blood, nutrients, gases, hormones, and wastes throughout the body. It entails the coordination of the heart, blood vessels, and blood to sustain and maintain homeostasis and cellular activity. (At resting condition body pumps blood around 5 liters /minute)

a. Heart: It circulates blood throughout the body. b. Blood vessels refer to the network of arteries, veins, and capillaries responsible for the transportation of blood. c. Blood: It function as a transport system for oxygen, nutrients, and waste materials.

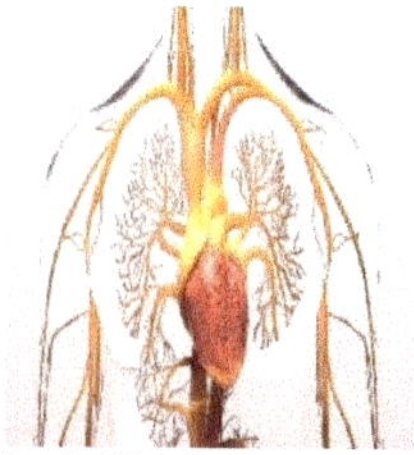

Fig. 4. Circulatory system.

iv. Respiratory system: The exchange of gases between the body and the environment is the responsibility of the respiratory system. It removes carbon dioxide, a waste product of metabolism, and oxygenates the blood. Which involves the exchange of carbon dioxide and oxygen (In a day human consumes 11,000 liters of air from atmosphere in which only 15-20% is oxygen).

a. Lungs: It enables the process of gas exchange, allowing for the uptake of oxygen and the release of carbon dioxide. b. The trachea and bronchi are the passageways that lead to the lungs. c. The diaphragm is a group of muscles that assist in the process of respiration. Inhaled CO, out exhaled exhalation

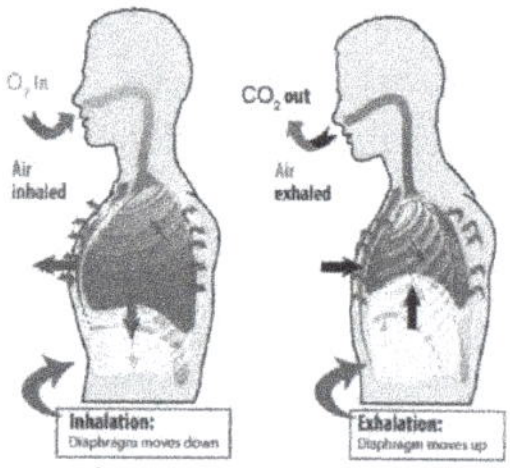

Fig. 5. Respiratory System.

v. Digestive system: Food is broken down into nutrients that the body can utilize for energy, growth, and repair during digestion. Additionally, it eliminates substantial debris from the body. (The entire digestive tract from mouth to anal canal of a healthy human adult is around 30 feets or about 9 meters long)

a. Mouth: The process of digestion commences with the mastication of food.
b. Esophagus is responsible for transporting food from the mouth to the stomach.
c. Stomach digests food by use of acids and enzymes.
d. Intestine: The small intestine is responsible for absorbing nutrition, whereas the big intestine reabsorbs water and rest eliminated as waste via. anal canal.
e. Liver, gallbladder, and intestines: They are responsible for the production and

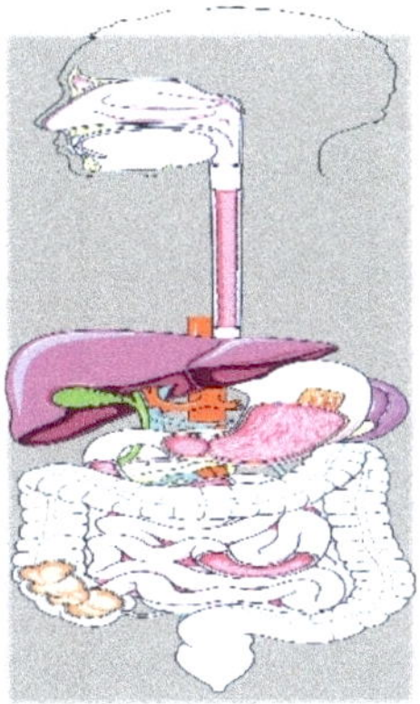

Fig. 6. Digestive System.

vi. Nervous system: Nerves are complex tissues that regulate and provide control over the body's responses to internal and external stimuli. It is accountable for the acquisition, processing, and transmission of information throughout the body. (About 86 billons neurons present in human brain as so far reported and around 120 million lost per hour in case of ischemic stroke)

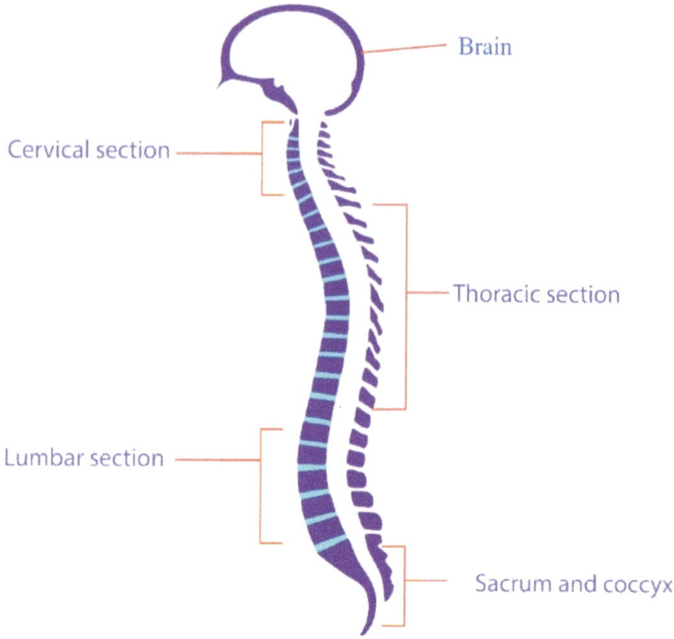

Fig. 7. Nervous System (Brain and spinal cord).

a. Brain serves as the central command center of the body.
b. Spinal cord facilitates the transmission of messages between the brain and the body.
c. Peripheral nerves are responsible for transmitting messages to and from the rest of the body.

vii. Endocrine system: The endocrine system is composed of tissues and organs that generate, accumulate, and eliminate energy from the body. These hormones are responsible for the regulation of a variety of bodily functions, such as metabolism, growth, development, neurological function, sexual function, reproduction, sleep, and mood. These are the contractile tissues responsible for regulating and executing the body's physiological processes. (There are total 8 endocrine glands in human body, these are also known as ductless glands)
a. Hormones are chemical substances that have the ability to regulate many physiological processes such as metabolism, growth, and development.

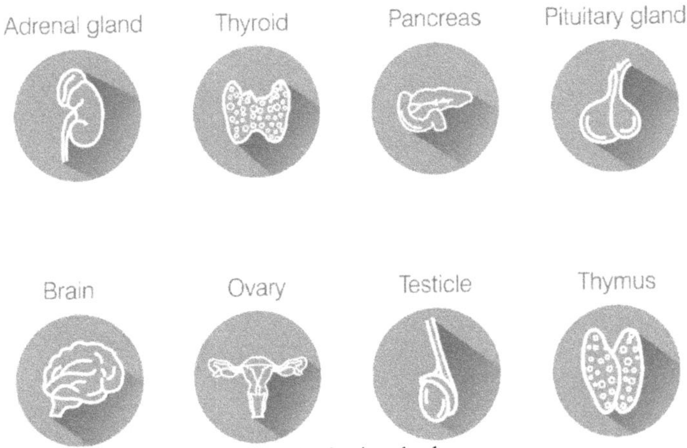

Fig. 8. Endocrine glands.

viii. Urinary system: The renal system, also referred to as the urinary system, is responsible for the regulation of blood volume and pressure, the excretion of waste and unnecessary substances from the bloodstream, the regulation of electrolyte and metabolite levels, and the maintenance of pH balance. (There are total 200liters of blood filter per day via. kidney)

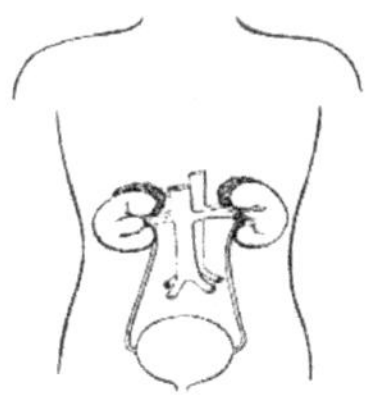

Fig. 9 Urinary system.

a. Kidneys: They perform the function of filtering and excreting waste products from the blood.
b. Bladder: It is the reservoir that holds water until it is eliminated from the body.
c. Ureter and urethra: It facilitate the passage of urine from the kidneys to the bladder and subsequently eliminate it from the body.

ix. Reproductive system: The genes required for reproduction are synthesized, stored, and transmitted by the reproductive system. They can preserve their genetic legacy by having offspring. This pattern encompasses a diverse array of organs and systems and is distinct between males and females.

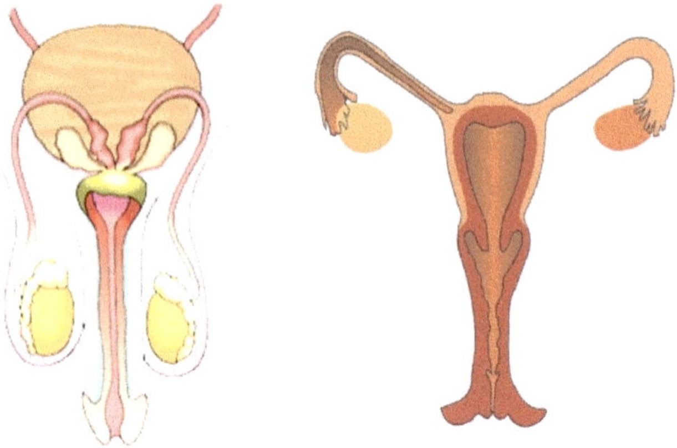

a. b.
Fig. 10. Reproductive System (a. Male and b. Female).

a. Male reproductive organs: It includes the testes, penis, and prostate gland.
b. Female reproductive organs: The female reproductive system includes the vagina and uterus, which are responsible for various reproductive functions.

x. Integumentary system: It is the body's outermost layer, which is responsible for thermoregulation, protection, and sensitivity. epidermis and adhesions.
a. Skin: It functions to insulate the body, control its temperature, and convey sensory information.
b. Hair and nails: Serves as an extra safeguards and aids for sensory functioning.

xi. Cells of the immune system: The immune system is a specialized cell that is crucial in safeguarding the body from infection, disease, and other harmful agents. These cells are a component of the immune system, which is a component of the body's defence system.
a. White blood cells: It serves the purpose of defending the body against diseases.
b. Lymphatic system: It is a network of glands and organs that aid in the removal of toxins and waste products from the body, it is divided into:
i. Lymph nodes: They are small, bean-shaped structures that are part of the lymphatic system.
ii. Blood vessels: Transport lymph away from the lymph nodes. And lymphatic veins transport lymph throughout the whole body.

1.1. Definition and scope of anatomy and physiology:

Anatomy refers to the study of the structure and organization of living organisms, including humans. It encompasses the examination of the many parts and systems that make up an organism. Scope, in this area, refer to the size, shape, and proportions of anatomical structures. Anatomy is a biological discipline that focuses on the examination of the structures and components of living creatures. This is a significant concern in the fields of biology and medicine, which specifically study biological systems. The word "anatomy" is derived from the Greek words "ana," meaning "up," and "tome," meaning "to cut." It specifically pertains to the process of dissecting the body in order to examine its components.

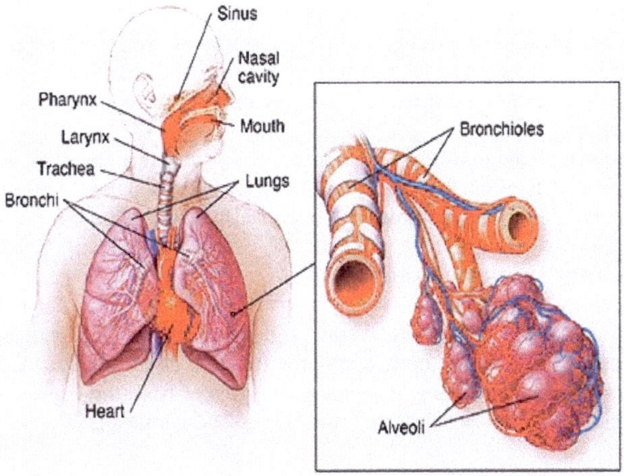

Fig. 11. Anatomy (Example: The structural part of respiratory system).

Cell dimensions or scope of anatomy:

i. Gross anatomy is the examination of the visible characteristics of the body without the use of a microscope, the following items are included:

a. Systemic Anatomy is the examination of distinct bodily systems, such as the cardiovascular or skeletal systems.

b. Regional Anatomy is the examination of distinct regions of the body, such as the head, neck, or belly.

c. Surface anatomy is the examination of the exterior structures of the body and how they are connected to the systems that lie underneath them.

ii. Micro-anatomy is the scientific examination of features that are only observable with a microscope, this includes:
a. Histology: It is the scientific examination of tissues.
b. Cytology: It is the scientific examination of cells.
Biochemistry: The study of the chemical processes and substances that occur within living organisms.

iii. Developmental anatomy: It is the scientific discipline that investigates the process by which an organism grows and matures, starting from the moment of conception, this encompasses:
a. Embryology, which is the scientific examination of the process of embryonic development from fertilization birth to the fetal stage.
b. Fetology: It is the scientific discipline that focuses on the examination and analysis of the developing fetus from the conclusion of its embryonic stage to the moment of delivery.
iv. Comparative anatomy: It is the study of the similarities and differences in the physical structure of different species. Additionally, it offers valuable information on evolutionary connections and adaptations.
v. Pathological anatomy: It often known as morbid anatomy, is the scientific discipline that focuses on the examination and analysis of structural alterations in tissues and organs affected by illness.

Physiology's definition and scope:
Physiology is the branch of biology concerned with the normal functioning of living organisms and their parts. It focuses on understanding how the body's systems function and interact to sustain life and health. The word "physiology" originates from the Greek words "physis," which means "nature," and "logos," which means "study."

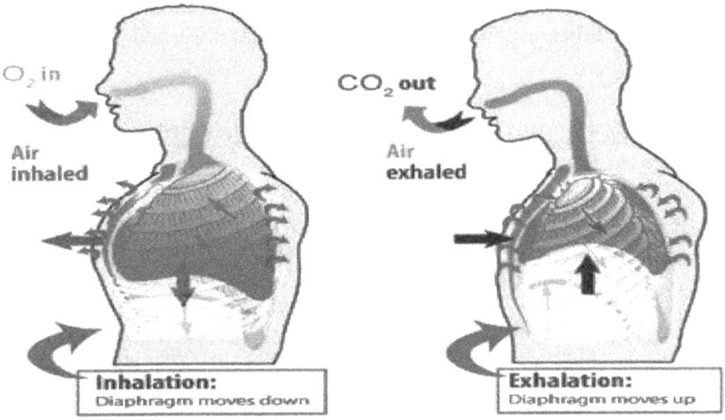

Fig. 12. Physiology (Example: The functional part of respiratory system).

Scope of physiology:

i. Cell physiology: The study of cellular functions, including pathways involved in cellular processes such as metabolism, signalling, and cell division.

ii. Organ System Physiology: It is the study of the function of specific organ systems, such as.

a. Cardiovascular physiology: Heart and blood vessel function.

b. Respiratory physiology: Lung and Airway Function.

c. Renal physiology: The mental body encompasses the functions of the mind and urinary tract.

d. Neurophysiology: The functions of the nervous system.

e. Endocrinology: the function of the endocrine glands and hormones.

iii. Comparative Physiology: The study of how different organisms perform similar functions and adapt to their environment.

iv. Environmental physiology/ Ecology: It is the study of how environmental factors such as temperature and altitude affect organism function.

v. Pathophysiology: It is the study of how disease or injury alters normal physiology.

vi. Exercise physiology: An examination of how exercise affects body functions, including cardiovascular, respiratory, and nervous systems.

Integration of anatomy and physiology:

Anatomy provides a description of the body's structure and explains how physiology makes these structures work, both disciplines are interrelated and essential to understanding the complexities of human physiology. For example, understanding the anatomy of the heart (its chambers, valves, and blood vessels) is essential to understanding its physiological role in blood pressure and blood vessel regulation, together, anatomy and physiology form the foundation of medicine, enabling healthcare professionals to better diagnose and treat diseases and conditions.

1.2. Levels of structural organization in the human body:

i. Chemical level

a. Molecules and Atoms: The most fundamental section pertains to the atoms (e.g., carbon, hydrogen, and oxygen) and molecules (e.g., water, proteins, and DNA) that constitute the basis of all entities.

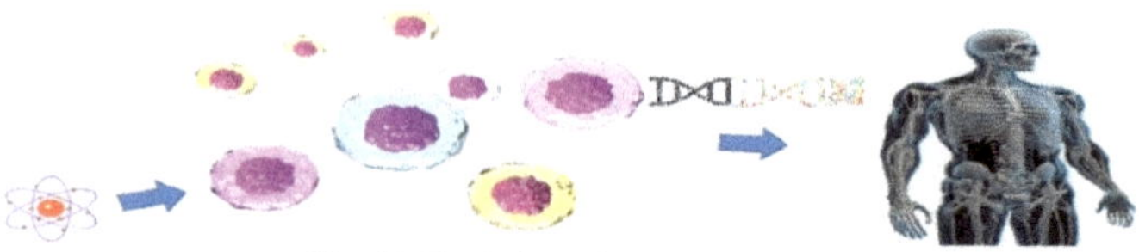

Fig. 13. Evolution of Human being.

ii. Cellular level

a. Cells: They are the smallest biological organisms in the body. Various functions are performed by various categories of cells, such as Nerve cell, stem cells.

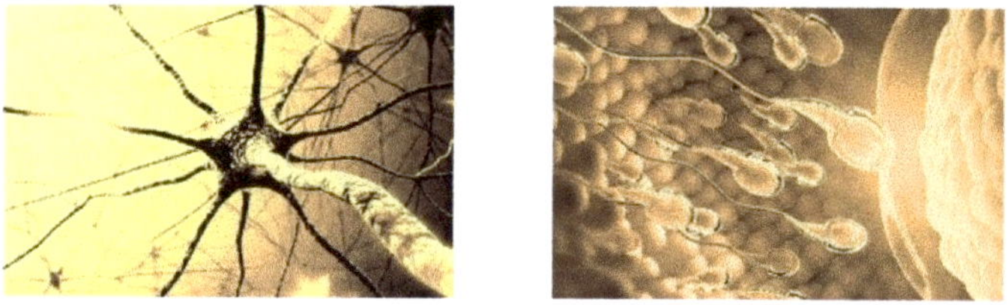

a. b.

Fig. 14. Cells (Examples: a. Neurons and b. Sperms)

iii. Tissue Level: Tissues are group of similar cell that plays a specific function, it is classified into four primary categories. i.e. Epithelial tissue, connective tissue, muscle tissue, nervous tissue in extent as an example the term elaborates nervous tissue is neurons they are clusters of cells that appear to collaborate in order to execute a particular function. i.e. in a neuron the cell body that carries signal from its axon region to dendrites of another neuron.

iv. Organ level

a. Organs: Those are structures that are composed of two or more types of muscles that collaborate to execute specific, intricate tasks, some examples are the brain, kidneys, lungs, and heart.

v. System level: Organ systems are collections of organs that share a common function. The human organism is composed of 11 primary organ systems:

a. Integumentary system: It provide insulation of the body, temperature regulation, and carries sensory information from one part to other part of the body those are all functions of the integumentary system. This encompasses cuticles, hair, and epidermis.

b. Skeletal System: It is responsible for the following functions those are the production of red blood cells, the promotion of movement, the storage of organic matter, the protection of internal organs, and the support of the body including bones and joints.

c. Muscular system: It is responsible for movement, posture and maintaining heat comprise the muscular system including bone marrow.

d. Nervous system: Nerves are responsible for the regulation of body activity, the processing of information through electrical signals, and the response to stimuli. This encompasses the nervous system, spinal cord, and brain.

e. Endocrine system: Hormones are utilized by the endocrine system to regulate bodily functions, these glands consist of the thyroid, pancreas, and adrenal glands.

f. Cardiovascular system: It is responsible for the transportation of nutrients, gases, hormones, and waste products throughout the body, including the heart and blood vessels are among them.

g. Lymphatic System: It is responsible for the recirculation of tissue fluids back into the bloodstream, as well as the protection against infection and disease, this system encompasses the lymph nodes, lymphatic vessels and the spleen.

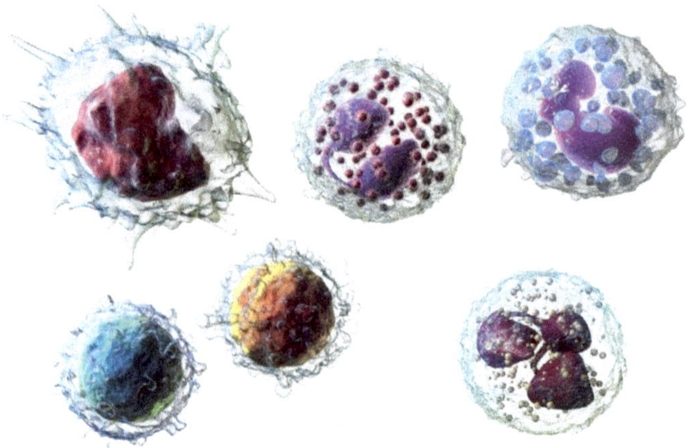

Fig. 15. Lymphatic cell.

h. Respiratory system: The process of supplying oxygen to the body and eliminating carbon dioxide is the responsibility of the respiratory system, the bronchial, tracheal, and nasal passages are among them.
i. Digestive System: It break the food, absorbs nutrients, and eliminates the wastes, with a series of steps called ingestion, propulsion, digestion, absorption and elimination. It includes the mouth, stomach, intestines, liver, and pancreas.
j. Urinary system: It is responsible for the removal of impurities from the blood, the regulation of blood pH, and the preservation of water balance in the kidneys, bladder, and urethra.
k. Reproductive system: It generates hormones and gametes (eggs and sperm) that induce the development of offspring, this includes uterus, fetus, and other associated structures comprise the reproductive system.

vi. Organismal level

a. Organism: The most advanced form of organization, in which all body systems collaborate to preserve the health and vitality of a living human being.

1.3. Basic life processes:

The human body, like all living organisms, generates numerous fundamental processes that are essential for the preservation and maintenance of homeostasis, these techniques consist comprising the following:

i. Cellular metabolism: A combination of all bodily chemical reactions, this process is classified into two primary categories.

a. Catabolism: Energy is released during the decomposition of solids into intractable forms.
b. Anabolism: Energy is required for the conversion of basic molecules into complex ones, a process known as anabolism.
ii. Responsiveness: The ability to recognize and respond to changes in the environment and beyond is exhibited, this encompasses the response to stimuli such as light, sound, temperature, and chemical signals.
iii. Movement: The entire body, individual organs, single cells, or intracellular components are capable of movement, this encompasses both voluntary movements (e.g., pacing, riding) and involuntary movements (e.g., pulse rate or peristalsis in the digestive tract).
iv. Growth and expansion: The body's or organs' girth increases as a result of the growth and proliferation of cells, an increase in cell number (hyperplasia) and an increase in cell size (hypertrophy) are both components of senescence.
v. Reproduction: The production and creation of a new individual, as well as the development of new cells for growth, repair, or replacement, takes place, this process guarantees the survival of species and the preservation of genetic continuity.
vi. Differentiation: The structural and functional specialization is achieved by the distinctions in undifferentiated cells, such as neurons, sperm and stem cells. Differentiation allows cells to execute particular functions within the organism.
vii. Excretion: The removal of metabolic waste, the body eliminates waste through channels such as the respiratory system (carbon dioxide), the digestive system (faecal matter), and the urinary system (uric waste in the form of urine).
viii. Homeostasis: In the event of external factors changing, homeostasis aims to preserve a consistent internal environment, in order to preserve a thin, optimal physiological state, homeostasis entails the regulation of factors such as pH, temperature, and electrolyte balance.

1.4. Homeostasis:

The process of homeostasis is the body's ability to maintain a consistent internal state in the face of fluctuations in external conditions, the proper functioning of cells, tissues, and organs is contingent upon this equilibrium. In order to regulate a variety of physiological processes, homeostasis necessitates the coordination of multiple systems.

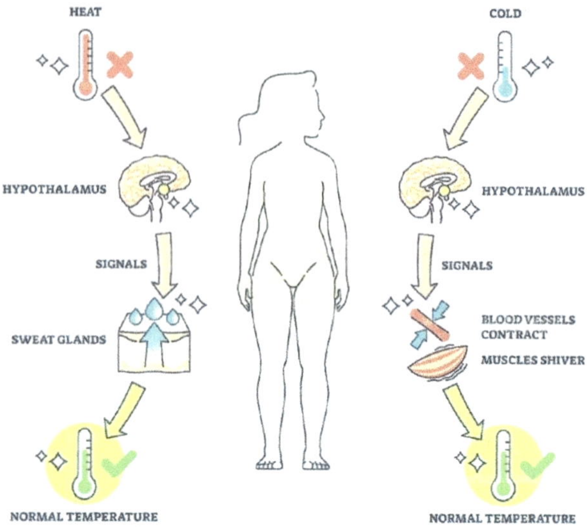

Fig. 16. Components of Feedback system.

The fundamentals of homeostasis:

a. Receptors: Those monitors the human body environment for any modifications or changes, whether they are internal or external. These variables they experience include blood glucose levels, blood pressure, and temperature.

b. Management of the control center: The brain or endocrine glands typically receive and process information from the receiver. The control center determines the appropriate response to maintain or restore equilibrium.

c. Effectors: The response indicated by the control center is executed by those who exert influence, the changes can be readjusted to a more favorable position by muscles, organs, or nerves.

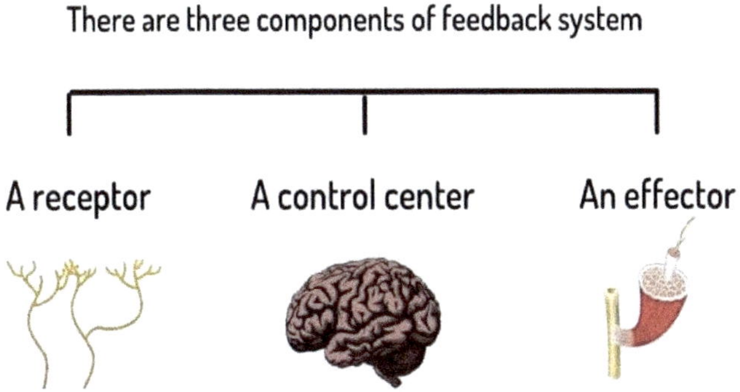

Fig. 17. Process of homeostasis.

Mechanism of homeostasis:

a. Negative feedback is facilitated by the mechanisms of homeostasis, those feedback are frequently carried out and its function to undo modifications in controlled environments for example, the body establishes mechanisms to regulate its temperature, including the production of perspiration. For instance, blood glucose monitoring insulin is secreted by the pancreas in response to an increase in blood glucose levels following a meal, insulin facilitates the absorption of glucose by cells, thereby reducing blood sugar levels. The pancreas releases glucose to elevate blood glucose levels when levels are insufficient.

b. Positive feedback those providing constructive changes in the body condition are at least partially influenced by these mechanisms, it is frequently employed by individuals to expedite the processes toward their conclusion, rather than to preserve equilibrium. For instance, blood clotting Platelets adhere to the affected area and emit significant quantities of platelet-attracting chemicals as a result of blood vessel damage, which leads to rapid haemorrhaging in order to halt the bleeding.

Examples of homeostasis:

1. Models of temperature regulation in homeostasis:

a. Receptor: Temperature fluctuations in the brain and epidermis are detected by thermometers.

b. Control center: The hypothalamus is responsible for the processing of information.

c. Effector: Variations in body temperature induce responses from sweat glands, muscles (vibration), and blood vessels (dilation or contraction).

2. Water equilibrium:
a. Receptor: The hypothalamus detects the osmoregulators in lacrimal glands and fluctuations in osmolarity of blood.
b. Control center: The secretion of diuretic hormone (ADH) is stimulated by the hypothalamus.
c. Effector: The kidneys regulate the reabsorption of water to optimize the osmolarity and volume of the blood.

3. Blood pressure regulation:
a. Receptor: Blood pressure fluctuations are detected by baroreceptors in blood vessels.
b. Control center: The processing of information by the medulla oblongata.
c. Effector: They regulate the size of blood vessels and the rate of heartbeat to maintain blood pressure.

The significance of homeostasis:
a. Survival: It ensures that the essential conditions for the survival and function of cells are maintained.
b. Health: It prevents diseases and disorders that result from imbalances, such as diabetes caused by improper glucose regulation.
c. Adaptation: The body is capable of adjusting to the escalating nature of environmental conditions, homeostasis is a dynamic process that is continuously adapting to internal and external changes in the body to maintain the optimal physiological environment for survival and function.

1.5. Basic anatomical terminology

Anatomical terminology provides a standardized language for describing the location and function of parts of the body, there are some fundamental terms and concepts:
Anatomical position: The standard reference position for the body in the study of anatomy. The body stands upright, facing forward, with arms at the sides, palms facing forward, and feet parallel.

Directional terms:
a. Superior (Cranial): Toward the head or upper part of the body; above, i.e. the head is superior to the abdomen.
b. Inferior (Caudal): Away from the head or toward the lower part of the body; below, i.e. the stomach is inferior to the lungs.
c. "Anterior (Ventral)" refers to the area in front of the body, i.e. the chest is anterior to the spine.

d. Posterior (Dorsal): Toward or at the back of the body; behind, i.e. the heart is posterior to the breastbone.
e. Medial: Toward or at the midline of the body; on the inner side, i.e. the nose is medial to the eyes.
f. Lateral: Away from the body's midline; on the outer side, i.e. the arms are lateral to the chest.
g. Proximal: Closer to the body part's origin or the point of attachment of a limb to the body trunk, i.e. the elbow is proximal to the wrist.
h. Distal: Farther from the origin of a body part or the point of attachment of a limb to the body trunk, i.e. the knee is distal to the thigh.
i. Superficial (External): Toward or at the body surface, i.e. the skin is superficial to the muscles.
j. Deep (internal): Away from the body surface; more internal, i.e. the lungs are deep in the rib cage.

Body plans and sections
a. Sagittal Plane: Divides the body into right and left parts.
b. Midsagittal (Median) Plane: Divides the body into equal right and left halves.
c. Parasagittal plane divides the body into unequal right and left parts.
d. Frontal (Coronal) Plane: Divides the body into anterior (front) and posterior (back) parts.
e. Transverse (horizontal) Plane: Divides the body into superior (upper) and inferior (lower) parts.
f. An oblique plane is one that passes through the body at an angle.

Body Cavities:
1. The dorsal body cavity divides into two subdivisions and protects the nervous system:
a. Cranial cavity: Encases the brain.
b. Vertebral (Spinal) cavity: Encases the spinal cord.

2. The Ventral body cavity divides into two subdivisions and the internal organs known as viscera.
a. Thoracic cavity: contains the heart and lungs.
b. The abdominopelvic cavity contains digestive organs, the urinary bladder, reproductive organs, and the rectum, it is further divided into:
i. Abdominal Cavity: Contains stomach, intestines, spleen, and liver.
ii. Pelvic Cavity: Contains urinary bladder, reproductive organs, and rectum.

<u>Regions of the Abdomen:</u>

1. Abdominopelvic Quadrants:
a. Right Upper Quadrant (RUQ)

b. Left Upper Quadrant (LUQ)
c. Right Lower Quadrant (RLQ)
d. Left Lower Quadrant (LLQ)

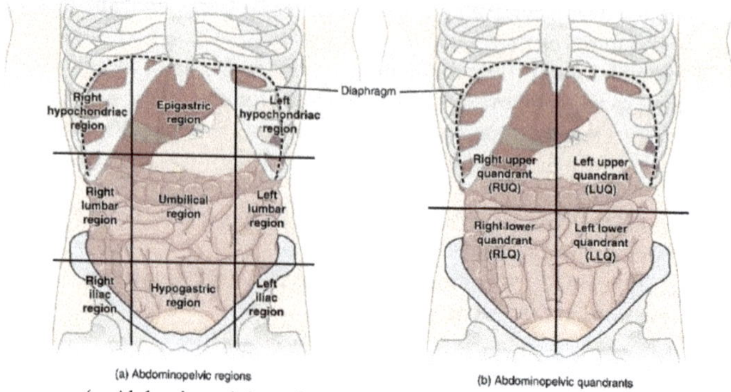

(a. Abdominopelvic regions and b. Abdominopelvic quadrants)
Fig. 18. Regions of the abdomen

Nine Regions:
1. Right Hypochondriac Region
2. Epigastric Region
3. Left Hypochondriac Region
4. Right Lumbar Region
5. Umbilical Region
6. Left Lumbar Region
7. Right Iliac (Inguinal) Region
8. Hypogastric (Pubic) Region
9. Left Iliac (Inguinal) Region

Other Key Terms:
a. Axial Region: Includes the head, neck, and trunk.
b. Appendicular Region: Includes the limbs (arms and legs).

Unit – 1.

Chapter 2.

Cellular level of organization

Cellular regulation is a foundational concept in biology that denotes the process by which cells organize and function as essential components of existence. The following is a synopsis of the points at the cellular organization level:

A. Definition of a cell: The fundamental nature of existence are cells, they are small organisms mostly capable of carrying out the essential functions that are essential for the existence of all life.

Structure and function: Each cell are designed with a specific layout that is appropriate for its intended purpose, this structure comprises the cytoplasm, genes, and cell membrane.

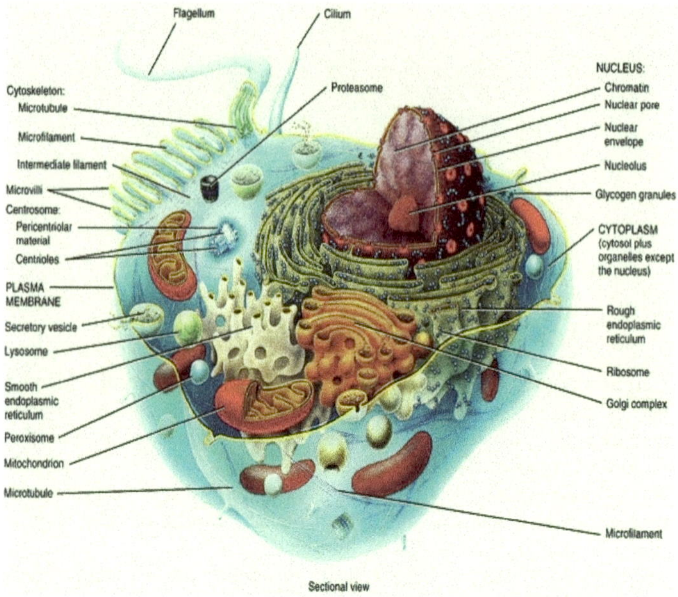

Fig. 19. Structure of animal cell.

B. Cellular types:

i. Prokaryotic cells: These are uncomplicated cells that lack a nucleus. Bacteria and fossils are two best examples.

ii. Eukaryotic cells: A nucleus and other membrane-bound organelles are present in eukaryotic cells, typical examples include protist cells, fungal cells, animal cells, and plant cells.

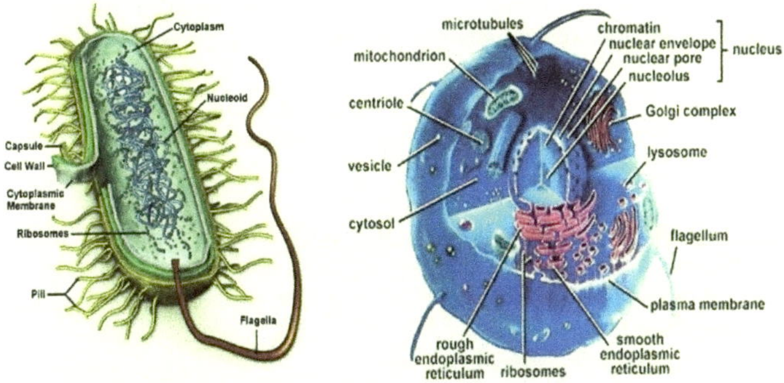

prokaryotic cell (bacteria)

eukaryotic cell (protists, fungi, animals, plants)

Fig. 20. Prokaryotic and eukaryotic cell.

C. Components of the cell:
i. Cell membrane: The movement in and out of cells is regulated by the lipid bilayer that constitutes the cell membrane.
ii. Cytoplasm: It is a jelly-like substance that is present in a cell and contains specific substances.
iii. Nucleus: The control center of a DNA-containing eukaryotic cell is the nucleus.
iv. Organelles: The components in the cell's primary parts including mitochondria (energy synthesis), ribosomes (protein synthesis), endoplasmic reticulum (protein and lipid synthesis), Golgi apparatus (sorting and packaging), and lysosomes (ground).

D. Cellular activity:
i. Metabolism: The chemical reactions that sustain the life of cells.
ii. Reproduction: Cells reproduce through processes such as mitosis (for growth and regeneration) and meiosis (for sexual reproduction).
iii. Stimulus response: Cells are capable of adapting to changes in their surroundings.
iv. Homeostasis is the process of preserving a consistent internal environment.

E. Cell structure in multicellular organisms:
i. Tissue: Groups of cells that appear to perform specific functions (e.g., Muscle tissue, nervous tissue).
ii. Organs: They are structures made up of various tissues, such as the heart and lungs.

iii. Organ system: groups of organs that work together to perform complex functions (e.g., digestive system, circulatory system).

F. Cell theory principles: All living things are made up of one or more cells, it is the basis of all living things. All cells come from pre-existing cells.

2.1. Structure and function of the cell: Human cells are highly specialized groups of structures (organelles) that perform specific functions essential for life, here is an overview of the main components and their functions:

I. Cell membrane (Plasma membrane):

a. Structure: Phospholipid bilayer embedded with proteins, lipids, and carbohydrates.

b. Function: It acts as a selective barrier, regulates the movement of substances into and out of the cell, and facilitates communication and signalling between cells.

II. Cytoplasm:

a. Structure: A gel-like substance composed primarily of water, salts, and proteins, filling the space between the cell membrane and nucleus.

b. Function: Supports and floats in organs and serves as a site for many cellular processes, such as metabolism.

III. Nucleus:

a. Structure: a large membrane-bound organelle containing chromatin (DNA and protein) and a nucleolus.

b. Function: Regulates cell functions through gene expression, maintains the genetic material of the cell, and affects cell growth, metabolism, and reproduction.

IV. Mitochondria:

a. Structure: Internal cristae are present in binary organs.

b. Function: It is to generate ATP through cellular respiration, which supplies energy for a variety of cellular functions.

V. Ribosome:

a. Structure: The ribosome is a structure composed of RNA and protein that is either associated with a dense endoplasmic reticulum or floats in the cytoplasm.

b. Function: The translation of mRNA into polypeptide chains is the process by which protein synthesis takes place.

VI. Endoplasmic reticulum (ER):
a. Structure: The fatty ER does not manifest a robust association with membranous tubes and pouch ER ribosomes.
i. Rough ER: It is responsible for the production and processing of proteins.
ii. Smooth ER: Facilitates the production of lipids, detoxifies compounds, toxins and stores calcium ions.

VII. Golgi apparatus:
a. Structure: A collection of slender outer sacs known as cisternae.
b. Function: Modifies, organizes, and binds proteins and lipids for storage or export from the cell.

VIII. Lysosome:
a. Structure: Organelles that are membrane-bound and contain aqueous enzymes.
b. Function: Through enzymatic decomposition, cellular debris, pathogens, and damaged organs are digested and recycled.

IX. Peroxisome:
a. Structure: Membrane-bound organelles that contain catalase and other enzymes.
b. Function: Detoxifies hazardous substances, such as hydrogen peroxide, and breaks down lipids and amino acids.

X. Cytoskeleton:
a. Structure: Protein filament networks, which encompass microfilaments, intermediate filaments, and microtubules.
b. Function: Aids intracellular transport, promotes cell migration, maintains cell morphology, provides structural support, and participates in cell division.

XI. Centrosomes and centrioles:
a. Structure: The centrosome is composed of two centromeres, which are circular structures composed of microtubules.
b. Function: Contributes to cell division, forms the mitotic spindle, provides cell structure, and forms microtubules.

XII. Vesicles:
Structure: Small, membrane-bound sacs.

Function: Transport materials within the cell and to the cell membrane for exocytosis.

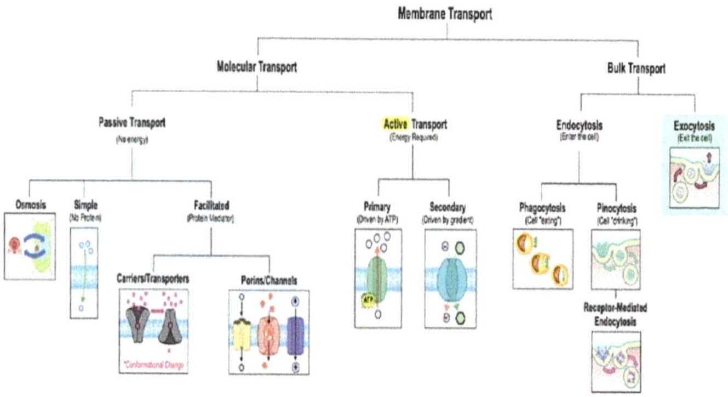

Fig. 21. Transport across cell membrane.

2.2. Transport across cell membrane: Transport is a critical mechanism that enables cells to interact with their environment, import nutrients, export waste products, and maintain homeostasis. There are numerous methods by which substances can pass through cell membranes:

A. Passive transport: It is low hill transport, contingent upon a concentration gradient and does not necessitate energy (ATP). This encompasses:

i. Simple diffusion: Its mechanism of action is straight forward and a lipid bilayer is directly penetrated by nonpolar particles, such as oxygen and carbon dioxide. The concentration gradient is the propelling force, which causes molecules to transition from higher to lower concentrations.

ii. Facilitated diffusion: Its mechanism of action is movement of specific transport proteins facilitate the movement of larger or polar molecules (e.g., glucose, ions) across the membrane, where it is enhanced concentration, hence channel proteins (which form apertures) and carrier proteins (which alter their conformation to become transport molecules) are associated proteins.

iii. Osmosis: Its mechanism of action is movement of water molecules through a selective permeable membrane, the driving force is the hydropotential gradient, the proteins that are involved are aquaporins, which are water channels.

B. Active transport: It is also known as up-hill transport, carriers that are currently operational in order to convey material against a concentration gradient, active transport necessitates energy (ATP), this encompasses:
i. Primary active transportation: Direct utilization of ATP to facilitate the transportation of molecules is the mechanism of action for instance, a sodium-potassium pump (Na^+/K^+ pump) that facilitates the exchange of Na^+ and K^+ within the cell.

ii. Secondary active transportation (cotransport): The energy of the electrochemical gradient that primary active transport induces is utilized by the mechanism, following types are:
a. Symport: The movement of two substances across the membrane in the same direction (e.g., glucose and Na^+).
b. Antiport: A mechanism in which two components move in opposed directions (e.g., Na^+/Ca^{2+} exchanger).

C. Bulk transport: It is the process of transporting small quantities of particles or fluids that necessitate energy, this encompasses:

<u>i. Metabolic endocytosis:</u> The mechanism of action for this substance is introduced into the cell through the formation of apertures by the intracellular membrane, which penetrates the cell's exterior and engulf the toxic and unwanted particles and destroy them, they are of 3 types:
a. phagocytosis is the process of "eating" cells, which entails the penetration of tiny particles or large cells.
b. Pinocytosis is the process of ingesting cells by imbibing extracellular fluid and dissolved solutions.
c. Receptor-mediated endocytosis: The formation of vesicles is induced by the interaction of specific molecules with receptors within the cell.

<u>ii. Exocytosis:</u> Engulf the extracellular material by forming vesicles that causes harm to the cell.
Structure: Vesicles containing endocytic material that are released from the cell after they fuse with the cell membrane.
Function: Secretes neurotransmitters, hormones, and digestive enzymes.

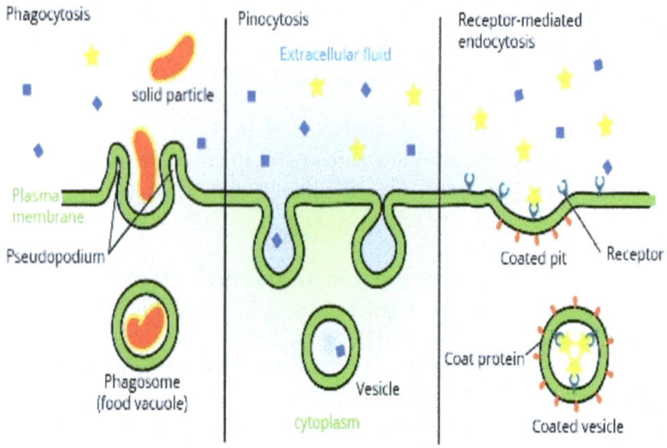

Fig. 22. Apoptosis.

D. Transmembrane proteins that are involved in the transportation process, these are of types

i. Channel proteins are hydrophilic channels that facilitate the diffusion of specific molecules or ions.

ii. Carrier proteins bind to specific molecules and endure conformational changes in order to transport them across the membrane.

iii. Protein pumps: Utilize ATP to facilitate the movement of ions or molecules as their concentration increases.

<u>2.3. Cell division:</u> The process of cell division are growth, development, and tissue repair are contingent upon human cell division, this involves the division of two or more genetically identical daughter cells and the replication of a single cell. In humans, there are two primary forms of cell division: mitosis and meiosis.

A. Mitosis: It is the process by which a somatic cell divides into two genetically identical offspring cells. Mitosis is essential for growth, tissue repair, and asexual reproduction. Mitosis comprises numerous phases:

<u>a. Interphase:</u>

i. G1 Phase: Protein synthesis and cell growth.

ii. S phase: DNA replicates, resulting in the production of two copies of each chromosome (sister chromatid).

iii. G2 phase: The cell continues to expand and prepare for mitosis.

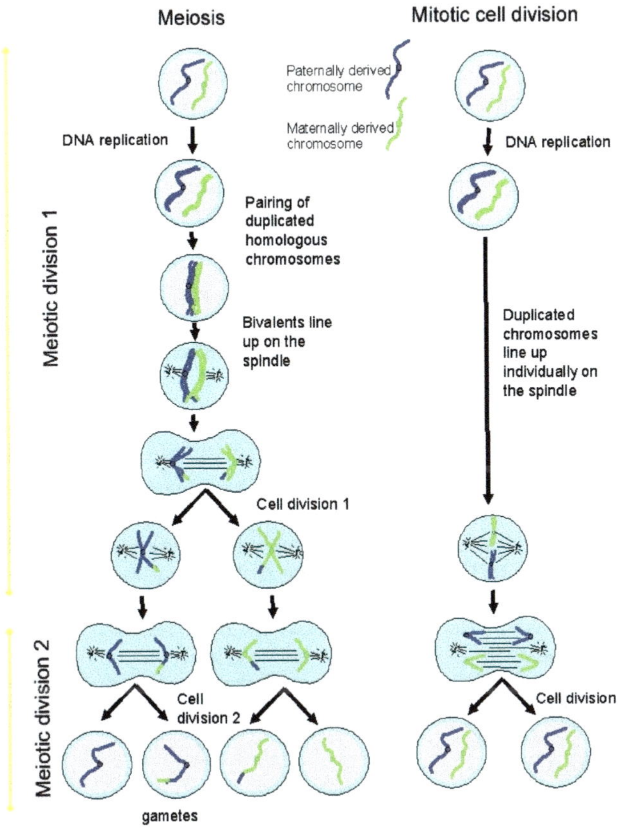

Fig. 23. Cell division (Meiosis and mitosis).

b. Prophase: Chromosome bands are formed by the assembly of chromatin, the process of atomic envelope decay commences, begin the formation and disintegration of a mitotic spindle that is composed of microtubules, the nucleus relocates to the cell's opposing poles in animal cells.

c. Metaphase: It is the equatorial plane of the cell. The nuclei of the chromosomes are attached by spindle fibers.

d. Anaphase: The (depravity) falling apart of sister chromatids are separated by spindle threads, which then direct them to the opposite poles of the cell.

e. Telophase: The chromatid reaches the poles and initiates additional disassembly into chromatin, around each chromosome, the nuclear envelope is rebuilt, the mitotic spindle undergoes division.

f. Cytokinin's (Cellular metabolism): Two distinct genetically identical daughter cells are produced as a consequence of the cytoplasm's division; this process is linked to cell division in animal cells.

B. Meiosis: It is the process within the organism in which the germ cells (embryos and ova) are generated, it produces four heterozygous cells from a diploid cell by reducing the number of chromosomes by half, meiosis is divided into two successive phases: meiosis I and meiosis II.

a. Meiosis I:
i. Prophase I: Homologous chromosomes duplicate and exchange genes through a process known as crossing over, the nuclear envelope has been collapsed, and a grinding mechanism has been established.
ii. Metaphase I: The metaphase plate is the site of the fusion of two parallel chromosomes.
iii. Anaphase I: The sister chromosomes remain attached, while the opposite poles attract homologous chromosomes.
iv. Telophase I: The chromosomes reach the poles, and the cells divide (cytokinesis) to produce two haploid cells.

b. Meiosis II:
i. Prophase II: In the organism the spindle apparatus in each haploid cell is rebuilt during the second prophase.
ii. Metaphase II: The metaphase plate is the location where the chromosomes are arranged during metaphase II.
iii. Anaphase II: Sister-chromatids migrate to opposite poles and separate.
iv. Telophase II: Chromatids remodel nuclear envelopes and reach poles, in this process of cytokinesis, four haploid cells are generated, each of which contains half the number of chromosomes present in the progenitor/ original cells.

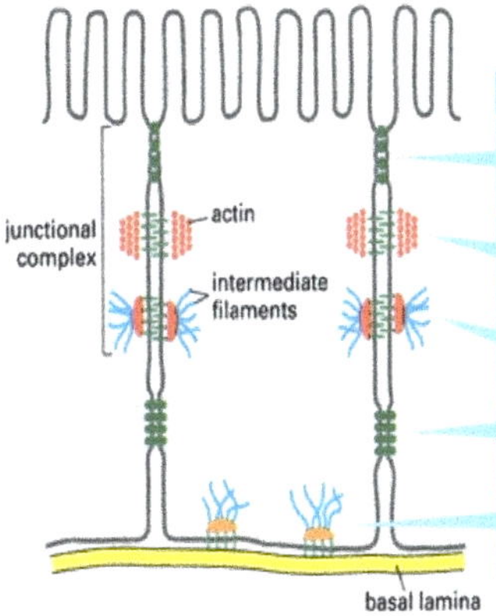

name	function
tight junction	seals neighboring cells together in an epithelial sheet to prevent leakage of molecules between them
adherens junction	joins an actin bundle in one cell to a similar bundle in a neighboring cell
desmosome	joins the intermediate filaments in one cell to those in a neighbor
gap junction	allows the passage of small water-soluble ions and molecules
hemidesmosome	anchors intermediate filaments in a cell to the basal lamina

Fig. 24. Cell junctions.

2.4. Cell junctions: Establishing connections between cells those are the specialized primary structures that establish connections between cells and the extracellular matrix. They are crucial in the preservation of tissue integrity, the facilitation of communication between cells, and the preservation of seamless flow. There are numerous varieties of cellular networks, each with its own unique structures and functions:

I. Tight junctions (Occluding junctions)

a. Structure: It is composed of proteins such as occludin and claudin, which collectively form a protective barrier around the cell surface.

b. Function: Develop a barrier that prevents molecules and ions from entering the intercellular space. Prevent the mingling of membrane proteins and lipids to preserve the distinct structure of the apical and basolateral surfaces.

II. Adherns junctions:

a. Structure: It involved in conventions cadherin proteins are formed by the attachment of actin filaments to the cytoskeleton by catenins.

b. Function: Develop a robust mechanical bond between adjacent cells, facilitate mobility and stability by connecting cell actin cytoskeletons to support membrane structure.

III. Desmosomes (Macula Adherents):

a. Structure: Consists of cadherin family proteins (desmogleins and desmocollins) that are connected to intermediate filaments (keratin) through desmoplakin and plakoglobin.

b. Function: Establish robust intercellular contact, particularly in tissues that are susceptible to mechanical stress, such as the epidermis and heart. It contributes to the preservation of muscle integrity by uniformly distributing mechanical energy within the cells.

IV. Hemi-desmosomes:
a. Structure: Adheres to the extracellular matrix, notably basement membranes, and contains integrins that are associated with intermediate fibers (keratin).
b. Function: Infuse the underlying tissue with endothelial cells to enhance its resistance to mechanical stress and increase its strength. The tissue structure can be supported by incorporating the cellular structure of the cell into the extracellular matrix.

V. Gap junctions (communicating junctions):
a. Structure: It composed of connexins that form channel called connexon proteins, which serve to distinguish between adjacent cells.
b. Function: Facilitate direct communication between cells by permitting the passage of ions, metabolites, and small signal molecules. It facilitates the coordination of cellular activities, such as the simultaneous contraction of smooth muscle cells and cardiac muscle.

2.5. General principles of cell communication:

Cellular communication is a fundamental mechanism through which cells perceive and respond to signals in their environment, this interaction is crucial for the preservation of homeostasis, the functions of different cell types, and cellular functions. The fundamental principles of cell communication are as follows:

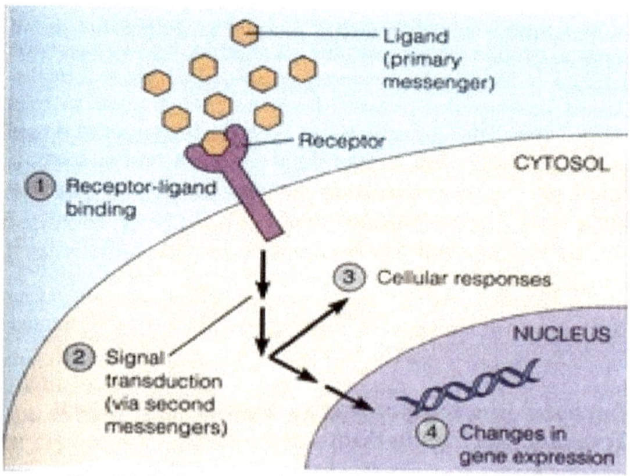

Fig. 25. Cell communication with those basic steps.

I. Signal reception: Signalling molecules (ligands) can be bound by specific receptors in the cytoplasm or surface of cells. Proteins or glycoproteins may serve as these receptors.

Types of receptors:
a. Cell surface receptor: External ligands (e.g., G-protein-coupled receptors, receptor tyrosine kinases) are bound by extracellular ligands, which are embedded within the cell.
b. Intracellular receptors: Those are located inside the cell, and bind to ligands that can cross cell membranes, such as steroid hormone receptors.

II. Signals transduction: The signal transduction pathway is activated by a conformational change that occurs when a receptor binds a ligand, polysaccharides and molecules with secondary messengers are typically involved in this process.
Second messenger: Minuscule(minute) molecules, such as cAMP, Ca2+, or IP3, that enhance intracellular signals, protein kinases are enzymes that phosphorylate target proteins, thereby modifying their activity (e.g., MAP kinases). Phosphatases are enzymes that neutralize symptoms by removing phosphate groups.

III. Signal amplification mechanism: The activation of numerous secondary or downstream proteins can result in signal amplification through ligand-receptor interactions, the objective of this mechanism is to guarantee that a limited number of signalling molecules within the cell can have a substantial impact.

IV. Cellular response: Signalling pathways are employed to prompt cells to react to particular stimuli, including modifications in gene expression, protein activity, or cell behaviour.

Type of responses: a. Gene expression: The activation or repression of specific genes, known as gene expression, can result in modifications to protein synthesis. b. Metabolic changes: Adaptation refers to the modification of metabolic pathways to accommodate the requirements of the cell. c. Cytoskeleton rearrangement: A modification in the size, motility, or distribution of a cell. d. Secretion of molecules: Molecular excretion is the process of removing cells, neurotransmitters, or other signalling molecules.

V. Signal termination: Cells possess mechanisms to terminate signalling in order to prevent excessive stimulation, these consist of the removal of second messengers, the inactivation of receptors, and the disruption of signalling molecules, it guarantees that the duration and intensity of the cellular response are suitable.

VI. Types of cell signalling:
a. Autocrine signalling is the process by which cells respond to signals that they have produced themselves.
b. Paracrine signalling: The signals that are emitted by one cell have an impact on the cells that are located in close proximity.
c. Endocrine signalling: Hormones are released by the bloodstream, which affects peripheral cells.
d. Juxtracrine signalling: It necessitates direct cell-to-cell contact in order to transmit signals to molecules that adhere to cell membranes.
e. Synaptic signalling: Neurotransmitters are released by neurons in synapses to transmit signals to target cells in synaptic signalling.

2.6. Intracellular signalling pathways are activated by extracellular signalling molecules:

Intracellular signalling pathways are intricate circuits that convert extracellular signals into cellular responses, this process typically entails the binding of an extracellular signalling molecule (ligand) to the cell surface receptor, which in turn triggers a series of intracellular events. this procedure is summarized below.

I. Signal reception:
a. Extracellular signalling molecule: This may be a hormone, growth factor, neurotransmitter, or other signalling molecule.
b. Receptor binding: A specific receptor on the cell surface is the site of an extracellular signalling molecule's binding. Receptors, which are proteins, are typically internalized by the cell.

II. Activation of receptor:
a. Conformational changes: The receptor undergoes conformational changes as a result of the ligand's binding, which results in activation, types of receptors:
i. G-Protein-Coupled Receptors (GPCRs) activate G-proteins, which subsequently activate or inhibit other proteins, such as enzymes or ion channels. Upon ligand binding,
ii. Receptor Tyrosine Kinases (RTKs) dimerize and auto phosphorylate, thereby activating their kinase activity.
iii. Ion channel receptors: open or close in response to ligand binding, enabling the entry or exit of ions from the cell.

iv. Cellular receptors are typically located in the cytoplasm or nucleus and are capable of binding to hydrophobic ligands that diffuse through the cell, such as steroid hormones.

III. Signal transduction:
a. Second messenger: signal carriers, including cyclic AMP (cAMP), calcium ions (Ca^{2+}), and inositol triphosphate (IP_3).
b. Protein phosphorylation: Kinases phosphorylate target proteins, altering their function, this can amplify the signal and trigger a phosphorylation cascade. An example of this is the MAP kinase (Mitogen-Activated Protein Kinase) pathway.
c. Protein-protein interactions: Functional proteins interact with other proteins to transmit a signal.

IV. Amplifying the signal: Amplification mechanism of each activated amplification receptor can synthesize multiple second messenger molecules, and each kinase can phosphorylate multiple substrates, amplifying the initial signal, it ensures that a limited number of signalling molecules can elicit a critical cellular response.

V. Cellular response:
a. Gene expression: Activation or repression of specific genes by transcription factors, resulting in changes in protein synthesis.
b. Metabolic changes: Activation of enzymes that alter metabolic pathways,
c. cytostructural rearrangement: changes in cell size, motility, or division.
d. Secretion: Secretion refers to the release of signals by other molecules or hormones.
e. Cell survival or apoptosis refers to the pathways that lead to either cell survival or programmed cell death.

VI. Termination of the signals:
a. Deactivation of Receptors: It can either internalize, degrade, or recycle to the cell surface during inactivation.
b. Second messenger degradation: enzymes degrade second messengers (e.g., phosphodiesterase degrades cAMP).
c. Dephosphorylation: phosphatases remove phosphate groups from proteins, reversing the activity of the kinase. Example: Activation of a GPCR pathway
d. Ligand binding: In a cell, an extracellular ligand (e.g., adrenaline) binds to a GPCR.
e. G-protein activation: GDP is exchanged for GTP in the alpha subunit of the G-protein during G-protein activation.

f. Effector Activation: An effector protein (e.g., adenylyl cyclase) interacts with an activated G-protein subunit.
h. The second messenger production: Adenylyl cyclase catalyses the conversion of ATP into the second messenger, cAMP.
i. Protein kinase activation: cAMP activates protein kinase A (PKA). Specific target proteins are phosphorylated by PKA, which induces a cellular response (e.g., an elevated heart rate).

2.7. Forms of intracellular signalling: (Contact-dependent, paracrine, synaptic, endocrine): That occurs within cells Intracellular communication, which regulates a diverse array of cellular processes, is referred to as cellular signalling, a diverse array of molecular mechanisms is employed by cells to transmit signals from receptors to target molecules, the primary intracellular signals are as follows:

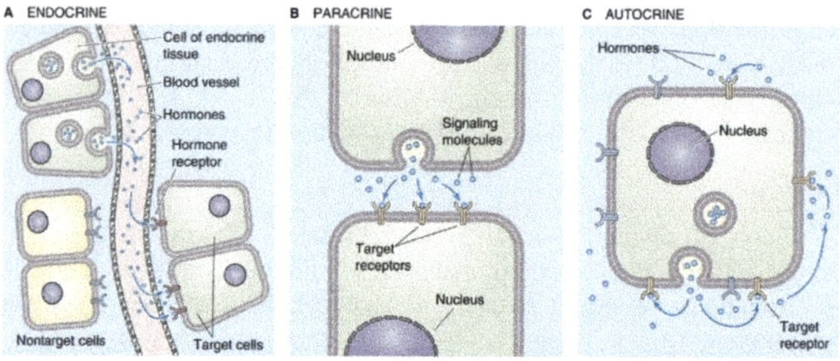

Fig. 26. Intracellular signalling.

I. Contact- dependent (Autocrine signalling) mechanism: The cell releases signalling molecules that bind to receptors on its surface, thereby initiating a response within the same cell, for example, cell growth factors have the ability to promote their own growth and proliferation.
II. Paracrine signalling mechanism: Signalling molecules are released by cells, which subsequently influence adjacent target cells in the local environment. Cytokines, which immune cells release to influence neighbouring cells, and neurotransmitters, which initiate the release of other neurotransmitters between nerve cells, are examples.
III. Endocrine signalling mechanism: Hormones enter the circulation and reach peripheral target cells throughout the body, example are the pancreas releases insulin, which regulates the movement of glucose into cells within the body.
IV. Juxtracrine transmission mechanism: Signalling molecules and membrane-bound receptors are typically involved in direct physical interactions that facilitate cell-to-cell communication. An illustration of

this is an interaction between immune cells, in which one cell presents an antigen on its surface to another cell.

V. Synaptic signalling mechanisms: Neurotransmitters are transmitted from neurons to target cells (such as other neurons, nerve cells, or neurons) through specific paracrine signalling at the synapse. For instance, muscle contraction is induced by the discharge of acetylcholine from nerve connective tissue.

VI. Intracrine signalling mechanism: Signalling molecules are activated within the same cell, as opposed to being released from it, for instance, steroid hormones bind to cellular receptors and influence gene expression within a cell.

VII. Direct signalling across gap junction's mechanism: The direct transfer of signal molecules and ions between neighbouring cells through gap junctions, which are channels that connect the cytoplasm of neighbouring cells, for instance, cardiac contraction is regulated by the flow of ions between cardiac muscle cells.

Forms of Intracellular signalling:

A. Communication-based intercellular signalling: **Contact-based intracellular signalling**, also referred to as juxtacrine signalling, is a form of cell communication in which the signal molecule remains affixed to the surface of the signalling cell and interacts directly with the receptor on a nearby target cell to facilitate muscle development, immune response, and cell differentiation.

Primary indicators and symptoms of direct communication between cells: The signal is transmitted by neighbouring cells through direct physical contact. Signalling molecules that are bound to the membrane: The ligand (signalling molecule) and the receptor are both anchored by the cell membrane. Only the cells that are immediately adjacent to the signalling cell are impacted by local signalling. Illustrations of communication-based signals are:

a. Immune communication antigen presentation:

Major histocompatibility complex (MHC) molecules are utilized by antigen-presenting cells (APCs) such as dendritic cells, macrophages, and B cells to present antigens on their surface. T cells initiate an immune response by recognizing these antigens through their T cell receptors (TCRs).

Action: Antigens are delivered to the TCR of T cells by APCs through MHC molecules, resulting in the activation of T cells and the subsequent immune response.

b. Signal of the notch developmental pathways:
The notch signalling pathway is indispensable for tissue growth and cell differentiation. Ligands and receptors: Delta, Serrate, and Jagged are ligands for the signalling cells, while Notch is the receptor for adjacent target cells.
Mechanism of action: The Notch receptor is proteolytically cleaved as a consequence of the ligand's binding to it. The intracellular domain of notch translocated to the nucleus and to modulate gene expression, thereby influencing the decisions of how cells will develop.

c. Nerves that are located within the interstitial direct cytoplasmic communication: Interstitial communication enables the direct transport of small molecules and ions between neighbouring cells, thereby facilitating coordinated cellular activities.
Structure: Connexin proteins establish networks by establishing connexins and establishing bridges between cells.
Function: Synchronizes the contractions of other muscles and unifies the contractions of cardiac muscle cells, signalling that is based on communication is crucial.
i. Accurate cellular response: This guarantees that the signal is only received by cells in direct contact, resulting in a highly localized and specific response. The fate of cells during embryonic development and tissue formation is significantly influenced by growth and differentiation. Immune surveillance facilitates the identification and response to pathogens or anomalous cells, as well as the maintenance of immune homeostasis.
ii. Methods of signalling that are founded on communication signalling: Membrane-bound ligands are expressed by signalling cells and interact with receptors on the surface of the target cell.
Signal transmission: The signal is propagated in the target cell by a structural change or cleavage that occurs when a ligand binds to a receptor.
iii. Cellular response: Intracellular signalling activates specific intracellular pathways, resulting in modifications to gene expression, protein function, or cell behaviour.

b. Paracrine intercellular signalling: Certain fundamental cells release their own cells, while other inner cells transmit the target code to distant cells and it influences his possessions primary indicators and symptoms.
i. Local signalling: Signalling molecules travel short distances to reach neighbouring cells.
ii. Non-hormonal: Consists of non-hormonal signalling molecules, including neurotransmitters, cytokines, and growth factors.

iii. Rapid response: The response is typically localized and rapid due to the brief distance of signal molecules.
iv. Paracrine signalling mechanisms: The discharge of signalling molecules of Paracrine factors (e.g., growth factors, cytokines) are released into the extracellular space by signalling cells.
v. Diffusion in target cells: These signalling molecules penetrate neighbouring target cells by diffusing through the extracellular matrix or interstitial fluid.
vi. Cell binding: Paracrine factors are bound to specific membranes on the surfaces of target cells. The activation of cell signalling pathways by ligand binding leads to modifications in cellular behaviour or function.

Target cells respond to signalling molecules in accordance with their functional pathways and characteristics. Models of paracrine signalling responsible for:
i. Growth factors: Factors that contribute to growth for instance, epithelial growth factor (EGF).
Function: EGF induces cell proliferation, differentiation, and growth in adjacent cells. Mechanism of action: EGF bonds to its receptor (EGFR) on neighbouring cells, initiating a signalling cascade that supports tissue repair and cell division.
ii. Cytokines: For instance, interleukins (e.g., IL-6).
Function: regulates inflammation and immunity. Interleukin is secreted by the immune system, and it acts on neighbouring immune cells to stimulate the immune system and modulate their function.
iii. Neurotransmitters: For instance, acetylcholine
Acetylcholine is responsible for the transmission of signals between nerve cells via nerve fibers.
The mechanism of action are as follows: Neurons on nerve cells bind to acetylcholine released by a muscle, resulting in muscle contraction.
iv. Signalling: Indications of desire Regulates cell fate, proliferation, and migration during the developmental process.
Method: Intracellular pathways that influence gene expression and cell behaviour are activated when Wnt proteins released by a single cell bind to Frizzled receptors on neighbouring cells.

The significance of paracrine signalling:
i. Tissue development and homeostasis: They are critical for processes such as cell growth, differentiation, and tissue repair in locally controlled environments.
ii. Immune response and communication: Accelerate the immune response by influencing local immune cells. Neuronal communication is crucial for the effective functioning of neurons, as it enables communication between neurons and target cells.

c. Synaptic cell signals: Synaptic intercellular signalling, a distinctive mechanism of cellular communication, takes place at synapses, where neurons connect with target cells, such as other neurons or nerve cells, to facilitate the integration of physiological mechanisms that facilitate rapid and precise communication within the nervous system, this symptom is significant.

i. Primary indicators and symptoms of signalling: The direct discharge of signalling molecules into target cells is initiated by synaptic junctions, drug transport is facilitated by neurotransmitters, which are chemical mediators that transmit signals across the synaptic cleft, the interaction between neurons and target cells is rapid and precise.

ii. Mechanisms of synaptic signalling: Action potential an actionable output, the action potential is somehow an electrical signal traverses the axon of the presynaptic neuron and enters the axon (presynaptic terminal).

iii. Neurotransmitter release: The release of an action potential triggers the opening of a voltage-gated calcium channel, which in turn releases calcium ions ($Ca2+$) into the presynaptic terminal.

iv. Exocytosis within synaptic vesicles that contain neurotransmitters is induced by this calcium release, resulting in their fusion with the presynaptic membrane.

v. Binding to receptors: Neurotransmitters bind to specific receptors on the postsynaptic cell membrane as they diffuse through the synaptic cleft.

These receptors can be:

a. When neurotransmitters bind to them, **ionotropic receptors**, which are ligand-gated ion channels, opens and enables the passage of ions across the membrane, which in turn transmits an electrical signal to the cell that is connected to the presynaptic receptor.

b. **Metabolic receptors** are G-protein-coupled receptors that can induce long-term alterations in cell function by activating cellular signalling pathways through second messengers.

c. Transmission of signals: Ionotropic receptors are capable of generating excitatory or inhibitory postsynaptic potentials (EPSPs or IPSPs) and directly mediate changes in membrane potential. Metabolism typically involves second messengers, such as cyclic AMP (cAMP) or inositol triphosphate (IP3), to initiate upstream cell signalling. This process results in delayed alterations and complicates cellular function.

d. Reuptake (Symptomatic relief or Neurotransmitter cessation): Transport proteins in the presynaptic neuron reabsorb neurotransmitters for recycling.

e. Enzymatic degradation: Neurotransmitters are degraded by enzymes in the synaptic cleft (e.g., acetylcholinesterase degrades acetylcholine).

Synaptic signalling models:
i. Excitatory stimulation in neurotransmitters: Glutamate AMPA or NMDA receptor the effect is characterized by the activity of glutamate ionotropic receptors, which generate an action potential in the postsynaptic neuron by depolarizing the postsynaptic membrane and producing sodium ions (Na^+).
ii. Obstruction of the nerves neurotransmitter: Gamma-aminobutyric acid (GABA). Receptor: GABA_A receptor.
Effects: GABA in result binds to ionotropic receptors, which generate chloride ions (Cl^-) and elevate the charge of the postsynaptic membrane. This reduces the likelihood of action potentials occurring in the postsynaptic neuron.
iii. Membrane Peptides: For instance, Substance P, the recipient is afflicted with rheumatoid arthritis, metabotropic receptors are frequently activated by neuropeptides. This triggers intercellular signalling pathways that modify the long-term excitability or plasticity of neurons or synapses.
Importance of synaptic signalling: Neuronal communication is essential for the transmission of information between neurons and other target cells, which in turn drives brain functions such as motor control, memory, and attention.

d. Endocrine intercellular signals: Endocrine-endothelial signalling is a method of cellular communication that enables signalling molecules, such as hormones, to infiltrate the bloodstream through endocrine glands and travel great distances to designated cells throughout the body, this signalling is crucial for the regulation of long-term physiological processes, such as growth, metabolism, and reproduction.

i. Long distance signalling: Proteins are transported from their production site to cells in remote regions of the body through the circulation.
ii. Systemic regulation: Hormones coordinate intricate physiological responses by influencing numerous tissues and organs.
iii. Hormone specificity: In order to guarantee that the hormone only impacts the appropriate cells, the target cells must possess a specific receptor.
iv. Endocrine signalling pathways in glands: The thyroid, adrenal, and pituitary glands are among the glands in the body that secrete hormones into the circulation.

v. Target cell internalization: Platelets traverse the circulatory system to reach target cells, in which hormones can be classified as: Peptide hormone: an amino acid (e.g., insulin), fatty acids in the circulation are the source of steroid hormones, including cortisol and estrogen.
Amino acid derivatives, including adrenaline and thyroid hormones, are produced from amino acids, i.e. adrenaline), cell binding is the process by which proteins adsorb to specific cells, either on the cell's surface or within it, peptide hormones and certain amino acid derivatives are prevented from crossing the cell membrane.
vi. Cell receptors: steroid hormone and thyroid hormone, which diffuse throughout the cell.

Transmission of signals:
A. Cellular receptors: Cellular signalling pathways are typically activated by binding, which typically involves second messengers such as inositol triphosphate (IP3) or cyclic AMP (cAMP). For instance, the binding of epinephrine to the beta-adrenergic receptor activates a G-protein, which in turn stimulates adenylyl cyclase to produce cAMP and activates protein kinase A (PKA).
i. Cell receptors: They directly influence gene expression by binding to components in the cytoplasm or nucleus, for instance, cortisol binds to its receptor in the cytoplasm and subsequently enters the nucleus to regulate gene transcription.
ii. Cellular Response: The binding of a hormone to its receptor initiates a sequence of cellular events that lead to a specific physiological response, such as fluctuations in metabolism, cell proliferation, or an immune response to disease activity.
iii. Eliminate the symptoms: Halt the hormone's activity, decomposed by enzymes in the liver or kidneys.
iv. Receptor internalization: This may encompass waste or recycling.
v. Feedback mechanism: Delivery mechanisms that prevent hormone synthesis regulate hormone levels.

Examples of endocrine transmission/ signalling:
a. Insulin: Pancreas is mainly associated for its generation, insulin receptor (tyrosine kinase receptor).
Effects: Promotes intracellular glucose transport by stimulating glycogen, thereby reducing blood glucose levels.
b. Thyroid hormones (T3 and T4). Thyroid gland is the source, thyroid hormone receptors (nuclear receptors) are receptors that influences gene expression to regulate metabolism, growth, and development.
c. Epinephrine: Adrenal medulla is the source, Beta-adrenergic receptors (G-protein-coupled receptors) are the receptors, that impact

induces a fight-or-flight response by elevating glucose levels, blood pressure, and heart rate.

d. Receptors for estrogen: Ovary (also produced to a lesser extent by other tissues), estrogen receptor (nuclear receptor) those are by modulating genes, the effect regulates reproductive function and secondary sexual characteristics, the significance of endocrine signalling its energy balance and metabolism are regulated by metabolic regulation, responsible for growth, development, and maturity.

e. Homeostasis: The internal equilibrium of a variety of physiological parameters, including blood glucose, calcium levels, and stress response, is maintained by homeostasis.

f. Reproduction: Fertility is the regulation of reproductive systems, including menstruation, pregnancy, and lactation.

Unit – 1.

Chapter 3.

Tissue level of organization

In multicellular organisms, the tissue level of organization is one of the fundamental tiers of biological organization. It denotes a collection of cells that share comparable structures and functions and collaborate to accomplish specific tasks. Tissues, which are essential for the structure and operation of organs and systems in the body, are composed of cells and their surrounding extracellular matrix.

Tissue classifications: In the human body, there are four principal categories of tissues, each with its own unique structure and function:

A. Epithelial Tissue:

Function: Forms glands, lines cavities and organs, that covers body surfaces and provide protective barrier and aids in the absorption, secretion, and sensations.

Characteristics: Cellularity is defined by the presence of a minimal extracellular matrix and tightly compacted cells; its polarity is defined by the presence of a basal (bottom) surface that is connected to underlying tissues and an apical (top) surface that is exposed to the environment or body cavity.

Avascular: Lacks blood vessels but receives nutrients through diffusion from underlying tissues.

Regenerative: Cells have the capacity to swiftly divide and replace damaged cells

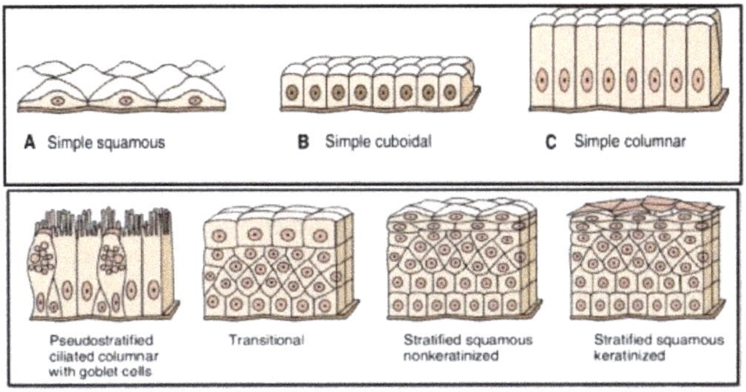

Fig. 27. Epithelial Tissue.

Types of epithelium cell include:

a. Simple epithelium: A single layer of cells, such as simple squamous, simple cuboidal, or simple columnar cells, is referred to as a simple epithelium.

b. Stratified epithelium: It consist of multiple layers of cells, such as stratified squamous, stratified cuboidal, and stratified columnar types.

c. Pseudostratified epithelium: A single layer with varying cell heights that appears layered (e.g., pseudostratified columnar).

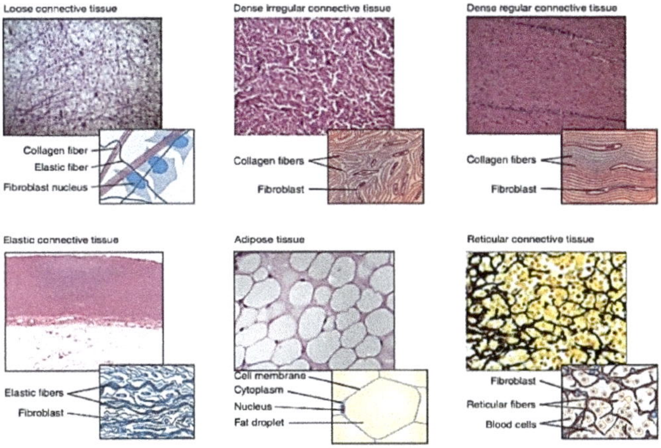

Fig. 28. Connective tissue.

B. Connective tissue

Function: Provides support, binds together, and safeguards organs and tissues. It offers metabolic and structural support.

Characteristics: Cell types consist of macrophages, adipocytes, and fibroblasts.

Extracellular matrix: Comprises fibrous substances (elastin, collagen) and doughy substances (gel-like substances), density of vascular tissue ranges from highly vascularized (e.g., bone) to sparsely vascularized (e.g., tendons).

Loose connective tissue: Areolar, adipose, and reticular tissue comprise loose connective tissue provides elasticity and support, elastic connective tissue includes both normal elastic tissue, such as muscles, and irregular elastic tissue, such as skin shows resistance and strength.

Specialized connective tissue: Bone, blood, and cartilage (including hyaline and elastic) comprise primary connective tissue, each serves a distinct purpose, such as supporting the body (bone) or transporting blood.

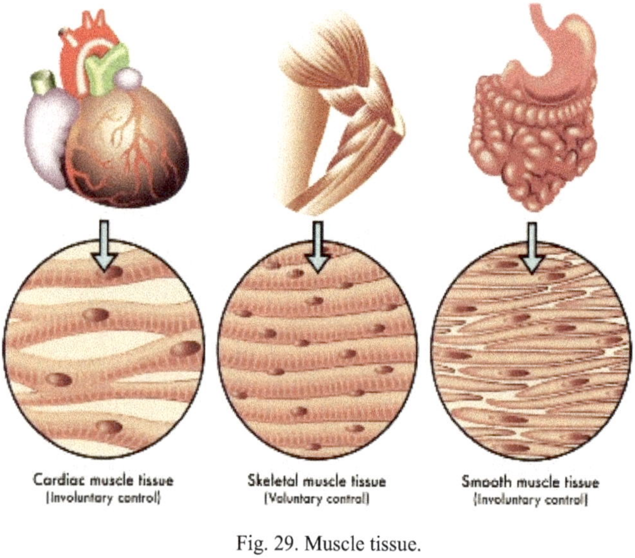

Fig. 29. Muscle tissue.

C. Muscle tissue: It is one of the functions of the muscle tissue is to facilitate the process of triggering by dragging impulses in voluntary and involuntary movements.

Muscles are accountable for both voluntary and involuntary movements.

Characteristics: Cellular Structure: Muscle cells are elongated and contain contractile proteins (myosin and actin).

Types of muscle tissue:

a. Skeletal muscles: they are attached to bones, contract and extend voluntarily, and aid in the movement of the body. B

b. Cardiac muscle: The presence of dotted, undesired cardiac muscles in the heart results in haemorrhage.

c. Smooth muscles, which are involuntary and non-striatal, are located in the walls of tubular structures (e.g., intestines, blood vessels) and are involved in functions such as peristalsis.

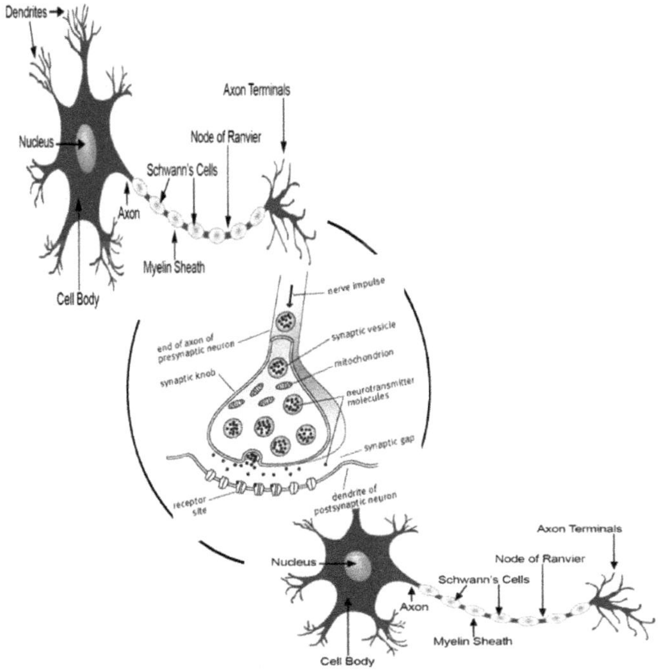

Fig. 30. Nervous tissue.

D. Nervous system: The nervous system's function is to transmit electrical signals throughout the body in order to regulate and control metabolism, it is involved in the processing of information, emotional arousal, and response.
Characteristics: Neurons include the functional cells that transmit electrical impulses, it consists of cell bodies, axons, and dendrites.

Neuroglia, which are also referred to as glial cells, are responsible for the maintenance of homeostasis, the provision of protective factors, and the support of neurons that includes astrocytes, oligodendrocytes, microglia, and schwann cells comprise these cells.

Structure: Axons, which are long horizontal fibers, are responsible for connecting various components of nerves.

Tissue function and interactions:
Formation of the organ: Tissues are composed, combined to form organs, each of which serves a distinct purpose, for instance, the stomach includes epithelial tissue (lining the interior), connective tissue (supporting structure), muscle tissue (enabling movement), and nervous tissue (regulating functions), which regulates different body activities.

Systemic function: The muscles collaborate to execute intricate physiological processes, for instance, the cardiovascular system consists of cardiovascular tissue (heart) and connective tissue (blood vessels) that are capable of pumping and circulating blood.

Classification of Tissues
Tissues are classified into four main types based on their structure and function, each type has distinct characteristics and roles within the body, detailed overview of each tissue type:

A. Epithelial Tissue
Function: Forms protective layers on body surfaces and organs, lines cavities, and is involved in absorption, secretion, and sensation.
Characteristics:
a. Cellularity: Composed of tightly packed cells with minimal extracellular matrix.
b. Polarity: Cells have an apical (top) surface and a basal (bottom) surface.
c. Avascular: Lacks blood vessels; nutrients are supplied by diffusion from underlying tissues.

d. Regenerative: High capacity for renewal and repair.

Types of epithelial tissues:

i. Simple Epithelium: Single layer of cells.

ii. Simple Squamous Epithelium: Thin, flat cells; involved in filtration and diffusion (e.g., lining of blood vessels).

iii. Simple Cuboidal Epithelium: Cube-shaped cells; involved in secretion and absorption (e.g., kidney tubules).

iv. Simple Columnar Epithelium: Tall, column-shaped cells; involved in absorption and secretion (e.g., lining of the digestive tract).

v. Stratified Epithelium: Multiple layers of cells.

vi. Stratified Squamous Epithelium: Multiple layers with the surface layer being flat; provides protection (e.g., skin surface).

vii. Stratified Cuboidal Epithelium: Multiple layers with surface cells being cube-shaped; involved in secretion (e.g., sweat glands).

viii. Stratified Columnar Epithelium: Multiple layers with surface cells being column-shaped; provides protection and secretion (e.g., parts of the male urethra).

ix. Pseudostratified Epithelium: Appears layered but is a single layer with varying cell heights; involved in secretion and movement of mucus (e.g., respiratory tract).

B. Connective Tissue

Function: Provides structural and metabolic support, binds tissues together, and stores nutrients.

Characteristics:

a. Cell Types: Includes fibroblasts, adipocytes, macrophages, and others.

b. Extracellular Matrix: Composed of fibers (collagen, elastin) and ground substance.

c. Vascularity: Varies from highly vascular (e.g., bone) to avascular (e.g., cartilage).

Types of connective tissues:

a. Loose Connective Tissue:

i. Areolar Tissue: Flexible and supports tissues and organs.

ii. Adipose Tissue: Stores fat and provides insulation.

iii. Reticular Tissue: Provides a supportive framework for organs (e.g., spleen, lymph nodes).

b. Dense Connective Tissue:

i. Dense Regular Connective Tissue: Parallel collagen fibers; provides tensile strength (e.g., tendons, ligaments).

ii. Dense Irregular Connective Tissue: Randomly arranged fibers; provides strength and support (e.g., dermis of the skin).

c. Specialized Connective Tissue:
i. Cartilage: Provides flexible support and cushioning (e.g., hyaline cartilage in joints, elastic cartilage in the ear).
ii. Bone: Provides rigid support and protection; involved in mineral storage and blood cell production.
iii. Blood: Transports nutrients, gases, and waste; involved in immune response and clotting.

C. Muscle Tissue:
Function: Facilitates movement through contraction, which can be voluntary or involuntary.
Characteristics:
a. Cell Structure: Elongated cells with contractile proteins (actin and myosin).

Types of muscle tissues:
i. Skeletal Muscle:
a. Characteristics: Striated and voluntary; attached to bones and responsible for body movement.
b. Structure: Long, cylindrical cells with multiple nuclei.

ii. Cardiac Muscle:
a. Characteristics: Striated and involuntary; found in the heart.
b. Structure: Branched cells with a single nucleus, interconnected by intercalated discs.

iii. Smooth Muscle:
a. Characteristics: Non-striated and involuntary; found in the walls of hollow organs (e.g., intestines, blood vessels).
b. Structure: Spindle-shaped cells with a single nucleus.

D. Nervous Tissue:
Function: Transmits electrical signals and processes information to control and coordinate body functions.
Characteristics:
a. Cell Types: Neurons: The primary functional cells that transmit electrical impulses, it consists of a cell body, dendrites, and an axon.
Neuroglia (Glial Cells): Support and protect neurons. Includes astrocytes, oligodendrocytes, microglia, and Schwann cells.
Structure: Neurons have long projections (axons) that connect different parts of the nervous system and communicate with other cells.

3.1. The structure, location, and functions of epithelial tissue are described:

Characteristics of endothelial cells include their structure, location, and functions, the epithelial tissue is a specialized tissue that envelops surfaces and lines cavities. It serves a diverse array of functions, such as sensing, protection, and traction. This section examines the layout, location, and specific functions of the endothelial tissue.

The structure of an epithelial cell consists of densely compacted cells with minimal extracellular matrix, including desmosomes, and complex junctions, which are cellular connective tissues that establish a secure connection between cells, the surface of internal cells exposes itself to the external environment or the lumen of an organ, it may possess specialized structures, such as microvilli or cilia.

Basal surface: A narrow layer of extracellular matrix and basement membrane connects the surface of endothelial cells to the underlying connective tissue.

Blood vessels: in the absence of blood vessels, the connective tissue beneath the surface disseminates nutrients and oxygen. The recycling power has a significant capacity for both renewal and maintenance.

Endothelial cells have the capacity to proliferate at a rapid pace in order to replace tissues that have been damaged or lost. A dense extracellular membrane in the lower extremity distinguishes the epithelial layer from the underlying connective tissue, regulating the exchange of molecules between the epithelium and connective tissue and providing structural support. The size and nature of the cells, along with their size and type, determine the classification of epithelial tissue.

The simple epithelium consists of one-dimensional cells, while the stratified epithelium consists of multi-layered cells, also known as the pseudo-stratified epithelium. The monolayer, while appearing stratified, displays a variance in cell length.

By cell shape:

i. Squamous cells are slender and flat, resembling scales; cube-shaped cells are shaped like cuboidal brackets; columnar cells are characterized by lengthy columns and tall structures.

The epithelium is smooth and squamous, with single-walled, slender cells.

Location: The pulmonary arteries make up the endothelium that lines blood vessels, including the heart. the glomeruli of the kidney.

Functions: a. It simplifies the process of filtering and passive diffusion; b. It guarantees frictionless circulation of lymph nodes and blood; it expedites the exchange of air, nutrients, and water.

ii. Simple cuboidal epithelium: The superficial cup- or cube-shaped cells that make up this epithelium have a straightforward cubic structure.
Location: The endothelium of the kidney. The thyroid gland and the surface of the ovary are examples of tissues of small size.
Functions: secretion and absorption. It creates a protective barrier for tissues; they play a role in the transportation of substances through the duct.

iii. The simple columnar epithelium is the smooth muscle in a column-shaped cell, i.e. the digestive tract, which stretches from the stomach to the duodenum, bladder fibroids, and fallopian tubes, contains single-walled, tall columnar cells.
Functions: include the elimination of water, the digestion of enzymes, and the absorption of nutrients (for example, in the intestines).

iv. Stratified squamous epithelium: This structure, which lubricates goblet cells, is characterized by a flattened posterior border and multiple lines.
Location: The epidermis covers the skin, the oral cavity, the oesophagus, and the uterus.
Functions: It is resistant to abrasion and friction. an infection-resistant barrier, it protects the underlying tissue from any mechanical damage.

v. Stratified cuboidal epithelium: Numerous layers make up the structure, with cup- or cube-shaped outermost cells.
Location: The musculature of the sweat ducts, the mammary glands, and the salivary glands.
Functions: It facilitates the secretion process and provides protection.

vi. The stratified columnar epithelium, also known as the stratified plain, conceals the exterior pillar in multiple sections.
The location includes portions of the male urethra, dryness of the conjunctiva, and some large ducts, such as salivary glands.
Functions: It offers hydration and protection.

vii. Pseudostratified columnar epithelium refers to columnar nuclei that undergo pseudo-stratification. Variations in cell height cause the appearance of strata, but there is only one layer.

Location: The upper respiratory tract and lungs comprise the structural lining of the trachea and the ducts of large glands.
Functions: These activities involve the absorption and movement of water, typically carried out by ciliates. In certain regions, these activities also serve as a form of protection and attraction.

3.2. The structure, location, and function of connective tissue:

Connective tissue is one of the four main types of tissues in the body, playing a crucial role in supporting, connecting, and protecting various tissues and organs.

Structure of connective tissue:
Connective tissue consists of three main components:
a. Cells: Different types of cells are present. i.e.
i. Fibroblasts: Produce fibers and ground substance.
ii. Adipocytes: Store fat.
iii. Chondrocytes are present in cartilage.
iv. Osteocytes: Found in bone.
v. Blood cells: Including red blood cells (erythrocytes), white blood cells (leukocytes), and platelets (thrombocytes).

b. Fibers provide support and strength to connective tissue.
i. Collagen Fibers: Strong and flexible fibers that provide tensile strength.
ii. Elastic fibers provide elasticity and allow tissues to return to their original shape after stretching.
iii. Reticular fibers form a supportive mesh in soft tissues such as the spleen and lymph nodes.

c. Ground substance: A gel-like material that fills the space between cells and fibers, providing a medium for nutrient and waste exchange. It consists of water, proteoglycans, and glycosaminoglycans.

Location of connective tissue: Connective tissue is found throughout the body and is classified into several types based on its structure and function:
a. Loose connective tissue:
i. Areolar Tissue: Found in the skin, mucous membranes, and around blood vessels and organs.
ii. Adipose tissue is located under the skin, around internal organs, and in bone marrow.
iii. Reticular tissue is found in lymphoid organs such as lymph nodes, spleen, and bone marrow.

b. Dense connective tissue:
i. Dense regular connective tissue is found in tendons and ligaments.
ii. Dense, irregular connective tissue is found in the skin's dermis, joint capsules, and organ capsules.
iii. Elastic connective tissue is found in the walls of large arteries and bronchial tubes.

c. A specialized connective tissue: (Cartilages and bones)
Cartilage: Found in joints, ear, nose, trachea, and intervertebral discs.
i. Hyaline Cartilage: Found in the nose, trachea, and ends of long bones.
ii. Elastic Cartilage: Found in the ear and epiglottis.
iii. Fibrocartilage can be found in intervertebral discs and knee menisci.

Bones form the skeleton.
Blood flows throughout the cardiovascular system.

Functions of connective tissue:
a. Support and Structural Framework: This provides a framework that supports and anchors tissues and organs in place. Bone and cartilage are key structural components.
b. Protection: Protects delicate organs. For example, the skull protects the brain, and adipose tissue cushions organs.
c. Insulation: Adipose tissue stores fat, which insulates the body and conserves heat.
d. Transportation: Blood, a fluid connective tissue, transports nutrients, gases, hormones, and waste products throughout the body.
e. Storage: Adipose tissue stores energy in the form of fat, and bone stores minerals like calcium and phosphorus.

Connective tissue plays a role in immune defence; blood contains immune cells; and reticular tissue provides a framework for lymphoid organs, it involves in wound healing and tissue repair. Fibroblasts produce collagen fibers that form a scar.

3.3. The structure, location, and functions of muscular tissue are described:

Muscular tissue is one of the four main types of tissues in the human body, along with epithelial, connective, and nervous tissues. It is responsible for movement and various vital functions within the body.

Muscle fibers, elongated cells specialized for contraction, make up the structure of muscular tissue. These fibers contain numerous myofibrils, which are bundles of actin and myosin filaments that slide past each other to produce contraction.

Classification of muscular tissue into three types based on its structure and function:
a. Skeletal Muscle:
Structure: Skeletal muscle fibers are long, cylindrical, multinucleated, and striated (having a striped appearance due to the arrangement of actin and myosin filaments).
Location: Attached to bones by tendons.
Function: voluntary movement, posture maintenance, and heat production. Skeletal muscles are under conscious control.

b. Cardiac Muscle:
Structure: Cardiac muscle fibers are branched, uninucleated (sometimes binucleated), and striated. Intercalated discs, containing gap junctions and desmosomes for synchronized contraction, connect them.
Location: Found exclusively in the heart's walls.
Function: Involuntary contraction to pump blood throughout the body. The heart's intrinsic conduction system regulates the rhythmic and automatic contraction of cardiac muscle, while the autonomic nervous system influences it.

c. Smooth Muscle:
Structure: Smooth muscle fibers are spindle-shaped, uninucleated, and non-striated.
Location: Found in the walls of hollow organs such as blood vessels, the gastrointestinal tract, bladder, and uterus.

3.4. The structure, location, and functions of nervous tissue are described:

As one of the four primary tissue types in the body, nervous tissue specializes in the reception, transmission, and processing of information.
Structure of Nervous Tissue
Neurons and glial cells make up the majority of the cells in nervous tissue.

I. Neurons: These are the primary functional cells of the nervous system responsible for transmitting information.

Neurons structure:
a. Cell Body (Soma): Contains the nucleus and organelles.

b. Dendrites: branched extensions that receive signals from other neurons or sensory receptors.
c. Axon: A long, single extension that transmits signals to other neurons, muscles, or glands. A myelin sheath may cover the axon, insulating it and accelerating signal transmission.
d. Synapses are junctions in which the axon terminals connect with other neurons or effector cells to transmit signals.

II. Neuroglia (Glial Cells): These cells provide support, protection, and nourishment to neurons.
Types of glial cells include:
a. Astrocytes: Maintain the blood-brain barrier and provide structural support.
b. Oligodendrocytes: Form the myelin sheath in the central nervous system (CNS).
c. Schwann Cells: Form the myelin sheath in the peripheral nervous system (PNS).
d. Microglia: act as phagocytes to remove debris and pathogens.
e. Ependymal cells line the ventricles of the brain and the central canal of the spinal cord, producing and circulating cerebrospinal fluid (CSF).

Location of Nervous Tissue:
The body contains nervous tissue in two primary locations:
I. Central Nervous System (CNS): Comprises the brain and spinal cord.
a. Brain: enclosed within the skull and divided into several regions, including the cerebrum, cerebellum, and brainstem.
b. The spinal cord extends from the brainstem down the vertebral column.

II. Peripheral Nervous System (PNS): Consists of all the neural elements outside the CNS.
a. Nerves: bundles of axons that extend to and from the CNS to the rest of the body.
b. Ganglia are clusters of neuronal cell bodies located outside of the CNS.

Nervous tissue functions
a. Sensory Function: Detects internal and external stimuli through sensory receptors and transmits this information to the CNS. This

includes sensations like touch, temperature, pain, and special senses (sight, hearing, taste, smell).

b. Integrative Function: Processes and interprets sensory input, stores information, and determines appropriate responses. This involves activities such as thinking, memory, and decision-making.

c. Motor Function: Sends signals from the CNS to effectors (muscles and glands) to produce a response. This includes voluntary movements (e.g., moving your arm) and involuntary responses (e.g., heart rate regulation).

d. Homeostasis: It maintains internal balance by regulating body processes such as temperature, blood pressure, and fluid balance.

e. Coordination and Control: Coordinates and controls body functions by sending and receiving signals to and from various body parts. This includes autonomic functions like digestion, respiration, and cardiovascular regulation.

f. Reflex Actions: They execute rapid, automatic responses to specific stimuli, such as pulling your hand away from a hot surface, through reflex arcs.

Related questions from unit 1

1. Describe the structure and function of cell membrane.
2. Elaborate the loose connective tissues.
3. Describe the structure and function of ribosome.
4. Describe in detail about the endocytosis process.
5. Describe the gap junction.
6. Define the structure and function of endoplasmic reticulum.
7. Explain in detail about lysosome.
8. Describe the process of formation of secondary lysosome.
9. Describe the synaptic signaling.
10. Explain the structure and function of peroxisome.
11. Write in detail about ribosome?
12. Explain the structure and function of histone.
13. Explain the structure and function of nucleus
14. Describe in detail about adipose tissue.

15. Describe in detail about peroxisome.
16. Explain briefly the secondary active transport.
17. Describe the passive transport mechanism.
18. Explain the term symport and antiport.
19. Write the structure and function of cytoplasm?
20. Describe the working of centrioles and chromosomes in human cell.
21. Explain nerve tissue with proper diagram.
22. Explain in detail the function of nerve tissues with structure.
23. Write the structure and functions of endoplasmic reticulum?
24. Explain the structure and function of microtubules.
25. Explain in detail about the 'power house of cell'.
26. Explain in detail rough endoplasmic reticulum with proper diagram.
27. Explain the structure and functions of plasma membrane.
28. Explain the cell cycle in human body.
29. Explain neurohumoral transmission with a label diagram.
30. Describe function of golgi bodies.

Unit – 2.

Topic	Page no.
Chapter 1: Integumentary system	60
1.1. Structure and functions of skin	62 – 63

Topic	Page no.
Chapter 2: Skeletal system	64 – 66
2.1. Divisions of skeletal system	66 – 68
2.2. Types of bone	68 – 70
2.3. Salient features and functions of bones of axial and appendicular skeletal system	70 – 78
2.4. Organization of skeletal muscle	78 – 79
2.5. Physiology of muscle contraction	80 – 81
2.6. Neuromuscular junction	81 – 82

Topic	Page no.
Chapter 3: Joints	83 – 85
3.1. Structural and functional classification of joints	85 – 86
3.2. types of joints movements and its articulation	87 – 88

Related questions from unit 2	89

Unit – 2.

Chapter 1.

Integumentary system

The body's interior structure is composed of organs and complexes that form the outer covering. The fundamental purpose of the body's protective system is to safeguard against external harm, and it significantly contributes to overall well-being and the maintenance of internal balance. The components of the integumentary system encompass:

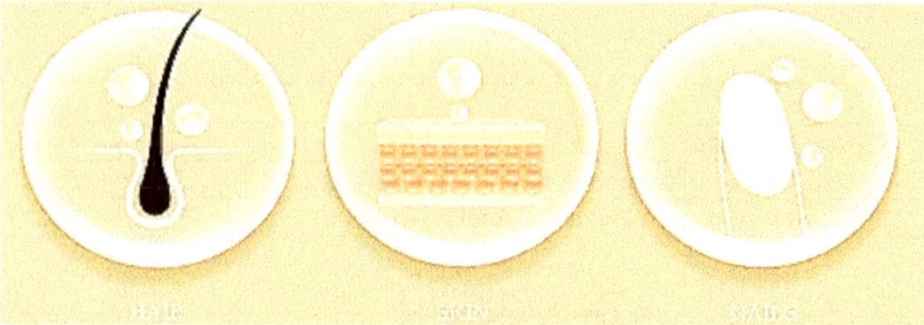

Fig. 31. Integumentary system.

a. The skin, including three primary layers, is the body's biggest organ.
i. The epidermis is the outermost stratum of the integumentary system, serving as a hydrophobic barrier and contributing to pigmentation.
ii. The dermis is situated underneath the epidermis and consists of thick connective tissue, hair follicles, and sweat glands.
iii. The hypodermis, also known as the subcutaneous layer, is the lowest layer of the skin.

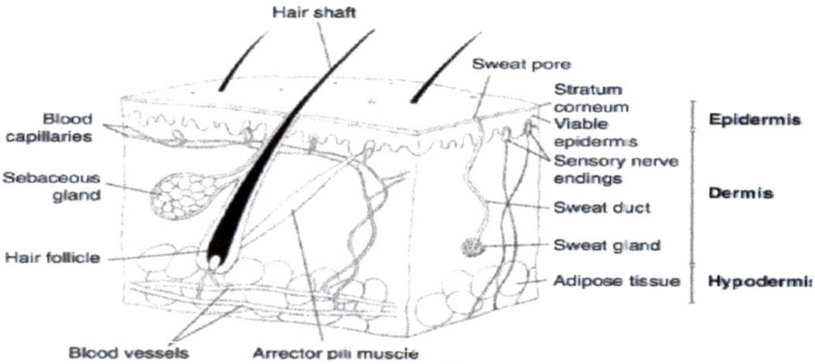

Fig. 32. Skin.

It is mostly made up of adipose tissue (fat) and connective tissue. Its main functions are to provide protection and elasticity to the body. Keratin, the substance responsible for the formation of hair, provides protection against ultraviolet (UV) radiation and assists in the regulation of body temperature through heat retention.
a. Nails: Nails are small, thin, dead cell of the body which elongates and protect the tip of fingers. Keratin also constitutes the structure of nails, providing protection to the fingertips and toes and enabling accurate movement.

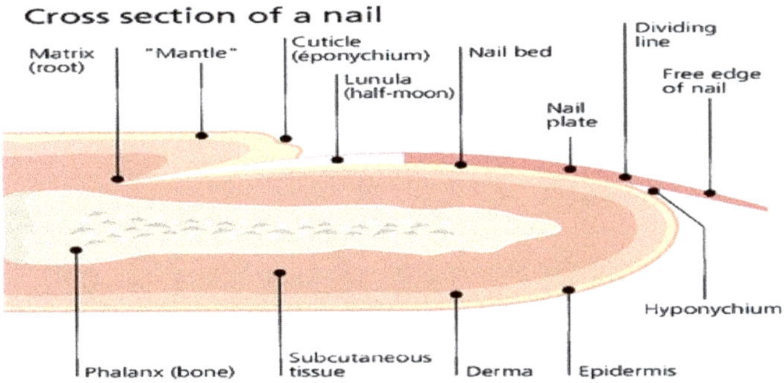

Fig. 33. Nails.

b. Glands:

i. Sebaceous glands are responsible for secreting sebum, an oily substance that helps maintain moisture in the skin and hair.

ii. Sweat glands are responsible for the production of sweat, which plays a crucial role in thermoregulation and waste elimination. Sensory sensitivity refers to the skin's ability to detect and respond to various feelings such as pressure, pain, and temperature, enabling the body to adapt to changes in the environment.

The functions of the integumentary system encompass:

i. Protection: Serves as a tangible obstacle against illness, toxins, and physical harm.

ii. Temperature: The regulation of body temperature is facilitated by the gut through the processes of sweat production and enhanced blood circulation.

iii. Sensation: The skin detects and transmits signals to the body, allowing it to perceive feelings such as heat, pain, and pressure.

iv. Excretion: Sweat glands facilitate the elimination of waste materials, including salt, water, and urea, from the body.

v. Vitamin D: Exposure to sunlight aids in the synthesis of vitamin D in the skin, which is crucial for maintaining healthy bones.

vi. Water resistance: The epidermis acts as a barrier, preventing excessive transpiration and maintaining proper hydration.

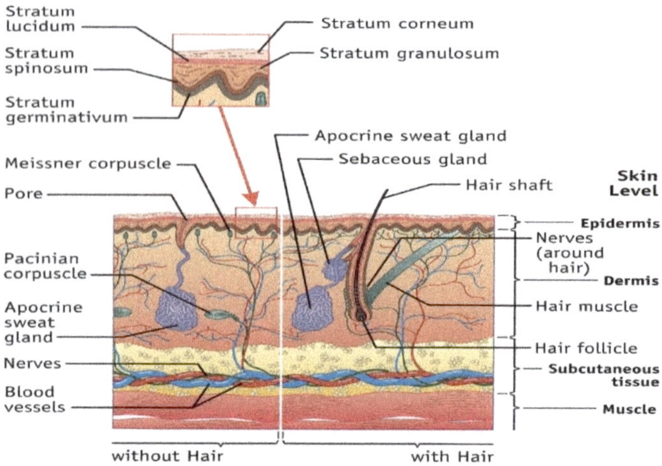

Fig. 34. Glands present in the layer of skin.

1.1. The structure and function of the skin:

The skin, being the biggest organ in the human body, acts as a crucial protective barrier and carries out several essential duties. Below is a comprehensive outline of its composition and operations. The physical manifestation of the outer layer of the body is the skin.

The skin is composed of three primary layers:

a. Epidermis: the outer layer it is the thin, outermost layer of the skin. It's primarily made up of keratinocytes, which produce keratin, a protein that helps waterproof and protect the skin.

i. Stratum Corneum: The outermost part of the epidermis consists of dead keratinized cells that constantly shed and are replaced by new cells from the lower layers.

ii. Stratum Basale: The deepest layer of the epidermis, where new skin cells are generated. This layer also contains melanocytes, which produce melanin, the pigment that gives skin its colour and protects against UV radiation.

b. Dermis: It is Middle Layer and its thicker than the epidermis and lies beneath it. It contains blood vessels, nerve endings, hair follicles, and glands.

i. Collagen and Elastin: The dermis is rich in collagen and elastin fibers, which give the skin its strength, flexibility, and elasticity.

ii. Sweat Glands: These glands produce sweat, which helps cool the body and excretes waste products.

iii. Sebaceous Glands: These glands secrete sebum, an oily substance that lubricates and waterproofs the skin and hair.
iv. Nerve Endings: The dermis contains sensory receptors that detect touch, pressure, pain, and temperature changes.
v. Hair Follicles: Structures that anchor the hair into the skin.

c. Hypodermis: (Subcutaneous Layer) It is the innermost layer that lies beneath the dermis and consists mainly of fat and connective tissue.
i. Fat Storage: This layer stores fat, which insulates the body, cushions internal organs, and serves as an energy reserve.
ii. Blood Vessels and Nerves: The hypodermis contains larger blood vessels and nerves that connect to the rest of the body.

Function of skin:
a. Protection: It serves as a tangible obstacle to protect against physical injury, disease-causing agents, and toxic chemicals. The presence of melanin in the skin provides protection against harmful ultraviolet (UV) radiation.
b. Thermoregulation: Perspiration and thermal energy aid in the process of bodily cooling. The blood arteries in the skin have the ability to dilate in response to heat or constrict to retain heat, so assisting in the regulation of body temperature.
c. Sensation: The skin possesses a diverse array of sensory receptors that detect pressure, pain, and temperature, enabling the body to react to alterations in the environment.
d. Excretion: The sweat glands present in the skin expel waste substances, such as salt, water, and urea, by means of perspiration.
e. Vitamin D: Sunlight exposure facilitates the production of vitamin D, an essential element for the absorption of calcium and the maintenance of bone health.
f. Water resistance: The outer layer of the skin, known as the epidermis, serves to prevent excessive water loss from the body, maintain proper hydration levels, and safeguard against dehydration.
The skin is an integral component of the body's immune system, housing specialized cells like Langerhans cells, which play a crucial role in identifying and combating infections.

Unit – 2.

Chapter 2.
SKELETAL SYSTEM

The skeletal system comprises of the structural framework of the body, consisting of bones, muscles, and joints. The human body relies on the skeletal system to provide support, protection, mobility, and to facilitate essential physiological processes.

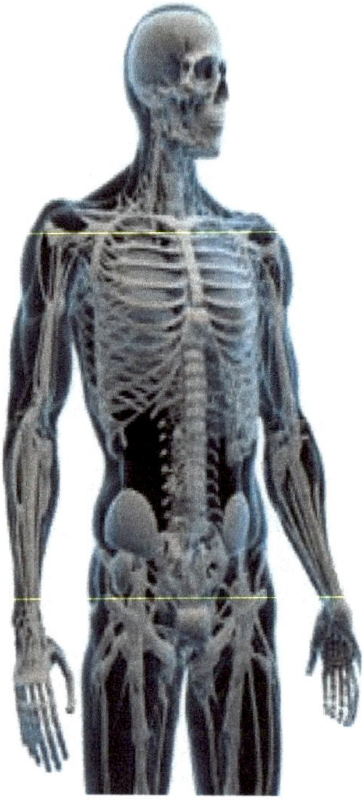

Fig. 35. Bones.

The structure of the skeletal system:
Bones: The human body contains a total of 206 bones, each with its own unique form and size that corresponds to its own purpose.

Types of Bones:
a. Long bones: They are located in the upper and lower limbs such as the femur and humerus, they reduce the weight and enhance movement.

b. Short bones: They are found in the wrists and ankles bones known as carpals and tarsals, having the ability for the stability and motion.
c. Flat bones: The skull, ribs, and spine are discernible as slender osseous structures, their function is to safeguard the internal organs and serve as an attachment site for tissues.
d. Irregular bones: Those bone is found in the spine and face. Their ideas are exceptional and have a distinct purpose.
e. Sesamoid bones: It possess tendon structures, including the patella, they provide protection to the muscles by preventing tension and injury.

Skeletal anatomy:
a. Compact bone: They are robust dense skeletal structure, they provide strength and support.
b. Spongy or Cancellous bone, often known as sponge bone: They possesses a permeable inner layer that is lightweight and comprises bone tissue.
c. Bone marrow: Those are located within the long bones, has the dual function of generating red and white blood cells as well as storing adipose tissue.
d. Cartilaginous bone: Fragile fibrous tissue located in the spaces between joints, ribs, ears, nose, and spine. It minimizes the resistance between the bones and dampens the impact of trauma.
e. Joints: Those contractions are anatomical connections between skeletal structures that facilitate movement.
There are several varieties of joints:
i. Synovial joints are characterized by their great degree of mobility, such as those found in the shoulder, hip, and knee.
ii. Cartilaginous Joints: Slightly movable joints like those between the vertebrae.
iii. Fibrous Joints: Immovable joints like the sutures in the skull.

Functions of the skeletal system:
i. Support: The skeletal system comprises the structural framework of the body, consisting of bones, muscles, and joints.
ii. Protection and movement: The skeletal system offers support, protection,
iii. Movement: Muscles are attached to bones, and when they contract, they pull on bones to produce movement.
iv. Mineral storage: Bones store minerals, particularly calcium and phosphorus, which can be released into the bloodstream as needed.
v. Blood cell production:
The bone marrow produces red blood cells, white blood cells, and platelets through a process called haematopoiesis.

vi. Energy storage: Yellow bone marrow stores fat, which serves as an energy reserve.
vii. Endocrine Function: Bones release hormones like osteocalcin, which helps regulate blood sugar and fat deposition.

2.1. Divisions of skeletal system:

The skeletal system is divided into two main divisions: the axial skeleton and the appendicular skeleton. Each division serves specific functions and consists of different bones.

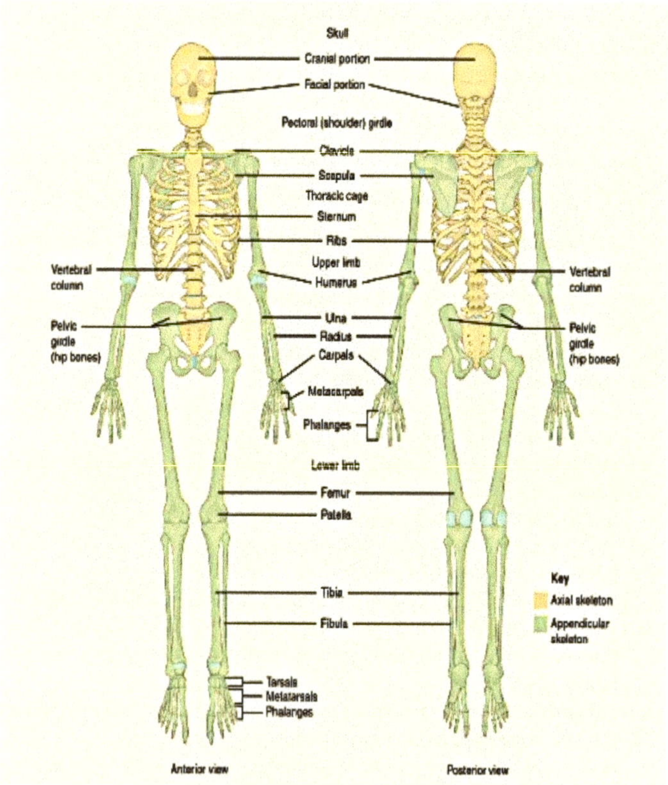

Fig. 36. Axial and appendicular skeleton system.

A. Axial Skeleton:

The axial skeleton forms the central axis of the body and includes bones that protect vital organs and support the body's structure.
Components:
a. Skull: Comprised of 22 bones (8 cranial bones and 14 facial bones), the skull protects the brain and forms the structure of the face.
b. Vertebral Column (Spine): Consists of 33 vertebrae divided into five regions:
i. Cervical (neck) - 7 vertebrae
ii. Thoracic (upper back) - 12 vertebrae
iii. Lumbar (lower back) - 5 vertebrae
iv. Sacral (pelvic region) - 5 fused vertebrae
v. Coccygeal (tailbone) - 4 fused vertebrae
vi. Rib Cage: Includes 12 pairs of ribs and the sternum (breastbone). The rib cage protects the heart and lungs and supports the upper body.
Hyoid Bone: A U-shaped bone located in the neck that supports the tongue and is associated with swallowing.

Functions:
a. Protection: Protects the brain, spinal cord, heart, and lungs.
b. Support: Provides a framework for the body and supports the weight of the head and trunk.
c. Attachment for Muscles: Serves as an anchor point for muscles involved in movement, posture, and breathing.

B. Appendicular Skeleton:
The appendicular skeleton includes the bones of the limbs and girdles that attach them to the axial skeleton, facilitating movement and interaction with the environment.
The following components are:
a. Pectoral (Shoulder) Girdle: Consists of the clavicles (collarbones) and scapulae (shoulder blades). It attaches the arms to the axial skeleton.

b. Upper Limbs:
i. Humerus: The upper arm bone.
ii. Radius and Ulna: The two bones of the forearm.
iii. Carpals: The 8 bones of the wrist.
iv. Metacarpals: The 5 bones of the hand.
v. Phalanges: The 14 bones of the fingers.
vi. Pelvic (Hip) Girdle: Formed by the hip bones (ilium, ischium, and pubis), it attaches the legs to the axial skeleton and supports the weight of the upper body.

c. Lower Limbs:

i. Femur: The thigh bone, and the longest bone in the body.
ii. Patella: The kneecap.
iii. Tibia and Fibula: The two bones of the lower leg.
iv. Tarsals: The 7 bones of the ankle.
v. Metatarsals: The 5 bones of the foot.
vi. Phalanges: The 14 bones of the toes.

Functions:
a. Movement: Provides the framework for movement by serving as attachment points for muscles.
b. Support and balance: Supports the weight of the body, especially when standing and walking.
c. Protection: Protects organs in the pelvic region.

2.2. Types of bones:

Bones in the human body come in various shapes and sizes, each designed to serve specific functions. Here are the different types of bones:

a. Long Bones:

Description: Long bones are longer than they are wide and have a cylindrical shape.
Structure: They consist of a shaft (diaphysis) and two ends (epiphyses). The shaft is composed mainly of compact bone, while the ends contain spongy bone with bone marrow.
Examples: Femur (thigh bone), humerus (upper arm bone), radius and ulna (forearm bones), tibia and fibula (lower leg bones), and phalanges (finger and toe bones).
Functions: Long bones support the weight of the body and facilitate movement by acting as levers.

b. Short Bones:

Description: Short bones are approximately equal in length, width, and thickness, giving them a cube-like shape.
Structure: These bones consist mainly of spongy bone covered by a thin layer of compact bone.
Examples: Carpals (wrist bones) and tarsals (ankle bones).
Functions: Short bones provide stability and support while allowing for some limited movement.

c. Flat Bones:

Description: Flat bones are thin, flattened, and usually curved. They have a broad surface area.
Structure: Composed of two parallel layers of compact bone with a layer of spongy bone in between.
Examples: Skull bones (like the frontal and parietal bones), sternum (breastbone), ribs, and scapulae (shoulder blades).
Functions: Flat bones protect internal organs (like the brain, heart, and lungs) and provide surfaces for muscle attachment.

d. Irregular Bones:
Description: Irregular bones have complex shapes that do not fit into the other bone categories.
Structure: They consist of a combination of spongy and compact bone.
Examples: Vertebrae (bones of the spine), sacrum, coccyx (tailbone), and certain facial bones like the mandible (jawbone) and sphenoid bone.
Functions: Irregular bones protect internal organs, provide support, and allow for complex movements.

e. Sesamoid Bones:
Description: Sesamoid bones are small, round bones embedded within tendons. They are found near joints.
Structure: These bones are usually formed in response to strain and have a smooth, rounded surface.
Examples: Patella (kneecap) is the largest sesamoid bone. Others are found in the tendons of the hands, feet, and knees.
Functions: Sesamoid bones protect tendons from stress and wear, reduce friction, and improve the leverage of muscles.

f. Sutural (Wormian) Bones:
Description: These are extra bone pieces that occur within a suture (joint) in the skull. Not everyone has them, and their number and location can vary.
Structure: Small and irregular in shape.
Examples: Found in the sutures between the flat bones of the skull, particularly the lambdoid suture.
Functions: These bones have no major functions but are considered normal anatomical variations.

2.3. Salient Features and Functions of Bones in the Axial and Appendicular Skeletal Systems:

The skeletal system is divided into two main parts: the axial skeleton and the appendicular skeleton. Each set of bones has distinct features and functions that are essential for various bodily functions.

I. Axial Skeleton

The axial skeleton forms the central core of the body and includes the skull, vertebral column, and thoracic cage.

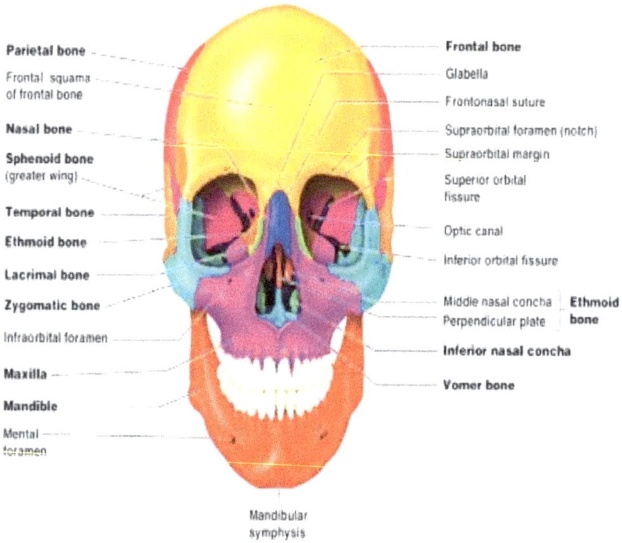

a. Front view

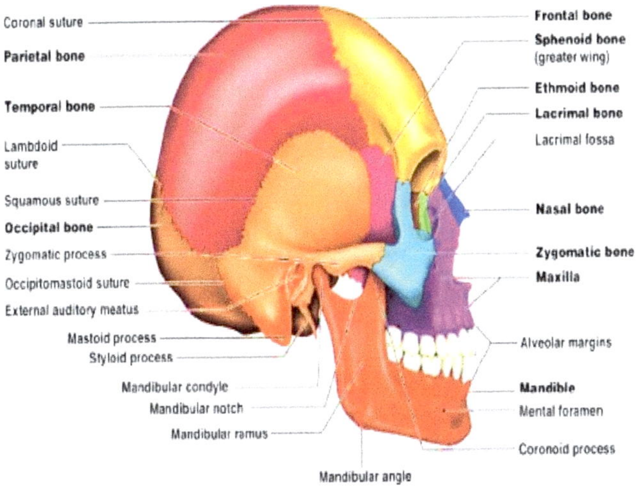

b. Side view

Fig. 37. Human skull.

A. Skull:

Salient features: It is composed of 22 bones (8 cranial bones and 14 facial bones), cranial bones include the frontal, parietal, occipital, temporal, sphenoid, and ethmoid bones. Whereas facial bones include the maxilla, mandible, nasal bones, and others.

Contains orbits (eye sockets), nasal cavity, and sinuses.

Function of skull:

a. Protection: Encases and protects the brain.

b. Support: Provides structure to the face and forms cavities for the sense organs (eyes, ears, nose).

c. Attachment points: Serves as an attachment site for muscles involved in chewing, facial expressions, and head movement.

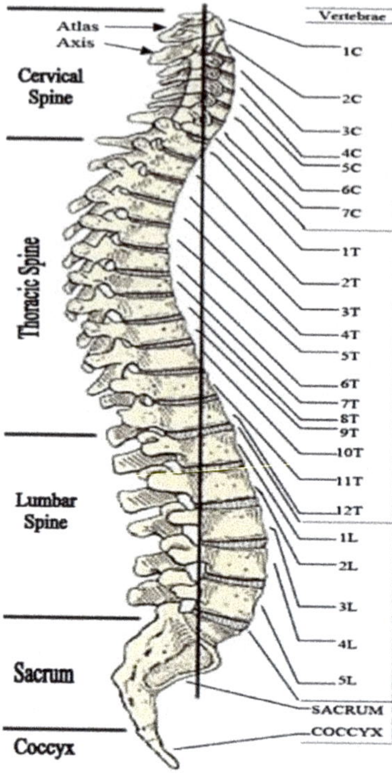

Vertebrae	Areas
1C	Blood supply to the head, pituitary gland, scalp bones of the face, brain, inner & middle ear, sympathetic nervous system
2C	Eyes, optic nerves, auditory nerves, sinuses, mastoid bones, tongue, forehead
3C	Cheeks, outer ear, face bones, teeth, trifacial nerve
4C	Nose, lips, mouth, eustachian tube
5C	Vocal cords, neck glands, pharynx
6C	Neck muscles, shoulders, tonsils
7C	Thyroid gland, bursae in shoulder, elbows
1T	Arms: elbow down; hands, wrist, fingers; esophagus and trachea
2T	Heart: valves and coverings, coronary arteries
3T	Lungs, bronchial tubes, pleura, chest, breast
4T	Gall bladder, common duct
5T	Liver, solar plexus, blood
6T	Stomach
7T	Pancreas, duodenum
8T	Spleen
9T	Adrenal and supra-renal glands
10T	Kidneys
11T	Kidneys, ureters
12T	Small intestines, lymph circulation
1L	Large intestines, inguinal ring
2L	Appendix, abdomen, upper leg
3L	Sex organs, uterus, bladder, knees
4L	Prostate gland, muscles of lower back, sciatic nerve
5L	Lower legs, ankles, feet
SACRUM	Hip bones, buttocks
COCCYX	Rectum, anus

Fig. 38. Vertebral column.

B. Vertebral column (Spine):

Salient features: It is composed of 33 vertebrae divided into cervical (7), thoracic (12), lumbar (5), sacral (5 fused), and coccygeal (4 fused) regions, intervertebral discs between vertebrae act as shock absorbers, curvature of the spine provides balance and flexibility.

Function of vertebral column:

a. Support: Supports the head and trunk, allowing upright posture.

b. Protection: Encases and protects the spinal cord.

c. Movement: Provides flexibility and enables bending, twisting, and other movements.

d. Attachment points: Serves as an anchor for ribs and muscles of the back.

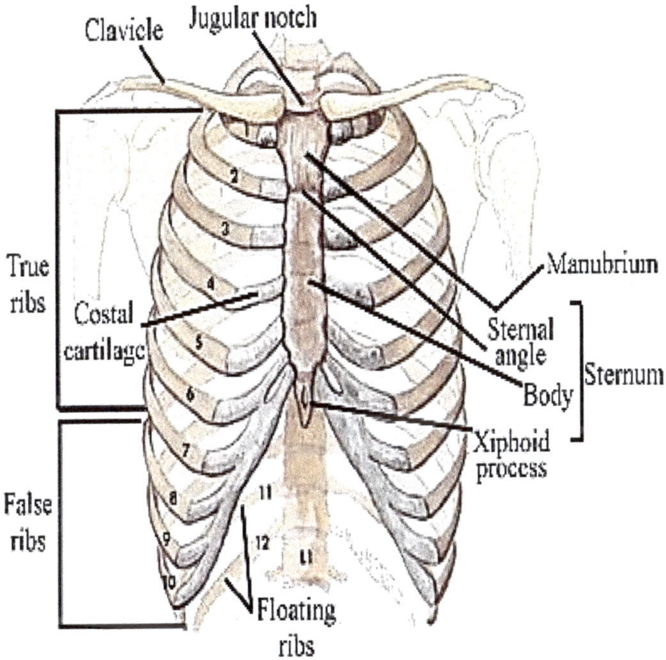

Fig. 39. Thoracic cage.

C. Thoracic cage (Rib cage):
Salient Features: It is composed of 12 pairs of ribs, sternum (breastbone), and thoracic vertebrae. True ribs (first 7 pairs) are directly attached to the sternum, false ribs (next 3 pairs) are indirectly attached, and floating ribs (last 2 pairs) have no anterior attachment.

Functions of thoracic cage:

a. Protection: Protects vital organs like the heart and lungs.

b. Support: Provides attachment points for muscles involved in breathing, shoulder, and upper limb movement.

c. Breathing: The rib cage expands and contracts during respiration to facilitate breathing.

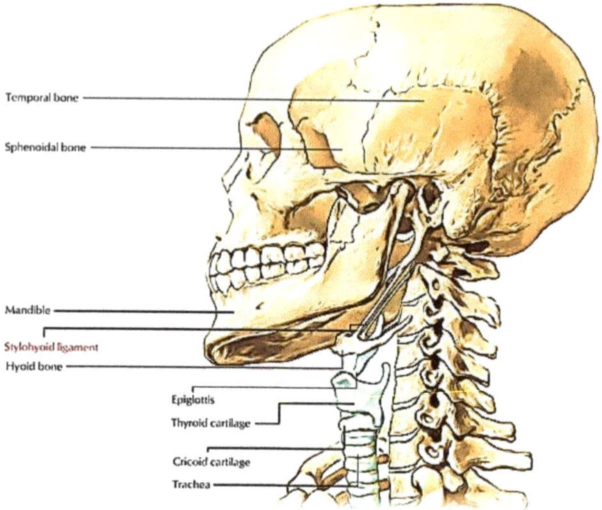

Fig. 40. Hyoid bone.

D. Hyoid bone:

Salient Features: A U-shaped bone located in the neck, not attached directly to other bones.

Function of hyoid bone:

a. Support: Supports the tongue and is associated with swallowing.

b. Attachment: Provides attachment points for muscles of the tongue, neck, and pharynx.

II. Appendicular Skeleton

The appendicular skeleton includes the bones of the limbs and the girdles that attach them to the axial skeleton.

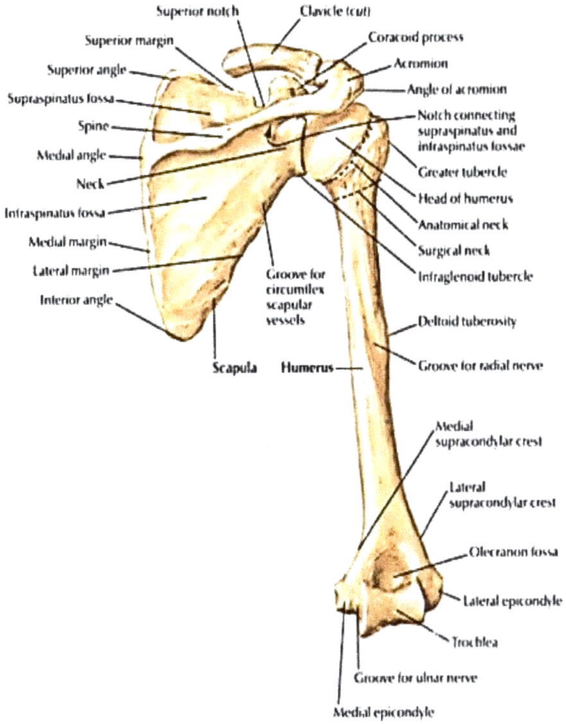

Fig. 41. Pectoral girdle.

A. Pectoral (Shoulder) girdle:

Salient Features: It is composed of the clavicles (collarbones) and scapulae (shoulder blades).

Function of pectoral girdle:

a. Support: Supports the arms and allows for their wide range of motion.

b. Attachment points: Provides attachment sites for muscles that move the arms and shoulders.

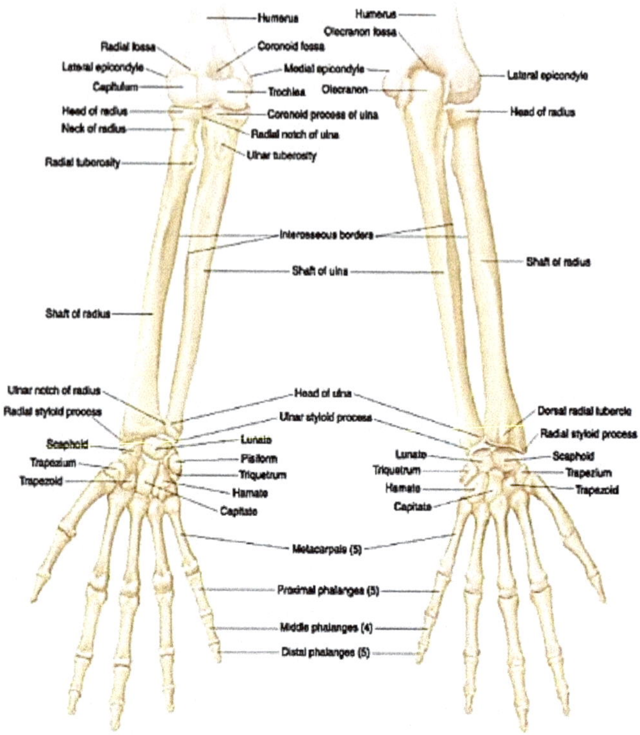

Fig. 42. Upper limb bones.

B. Upper limb bones:

Salient Features: It includes the humerus (upper arm), radius and ulna (forearm), carpals (wrist), metacarpals (hand), and phalanges (fingers).

Function of upper limb bones:

a. Movement: Enables a wide range of movements such as lifting, throwing, and grasping.

b. Support: Supports the weight of the upper body during activities like pushing or pulling.

c. Dexterity: Allows precise movements and manipulation, especially in the hands and fingers.

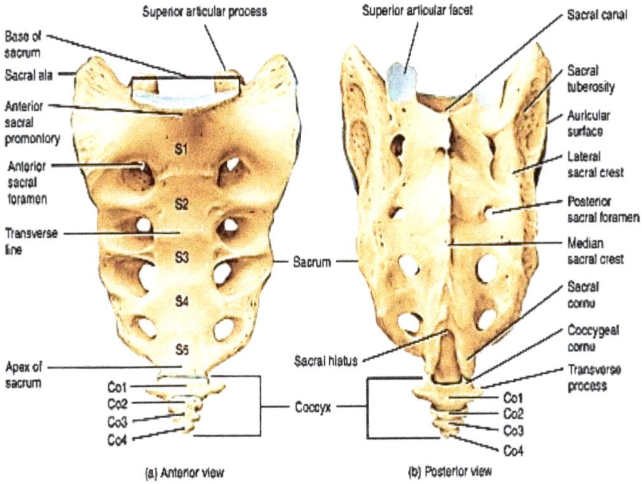

Fig. 43. Pelvic girdle.

C. Pelvic (Hip) girdle:

Salient Features: It is composed of the hip bones (ilium, ischium, and pubis), the pelvic girdle is more robust than the pectoral girdle to support the weight of the body.

Function of pelvic girdle:

a. Support: Supports the weight of the upper body and transfers it to the lower limbs.
b. Protection: Protects internal organs in the pelvic cavity, such as the bladder and reproductive organs.
c. Attachment points: Provides attachment sites for muscles involved in leg movement.

D. Lower limb bones:

Salient Features: It includes the femur (thigh), patella (kneecap), tibia and fibula (lower leg), tarsals (ankle), metatarsals (foot), and phalanges (toes), the femur is the longest and strongest bone in the body.

Function of lower limb bones:

a. Movement: Facilitates walking, running, jumping, and other movements.
b. Support and balance: Bears the body's weight, especially during standing and movement, also contributes to maintaining balance and posture.

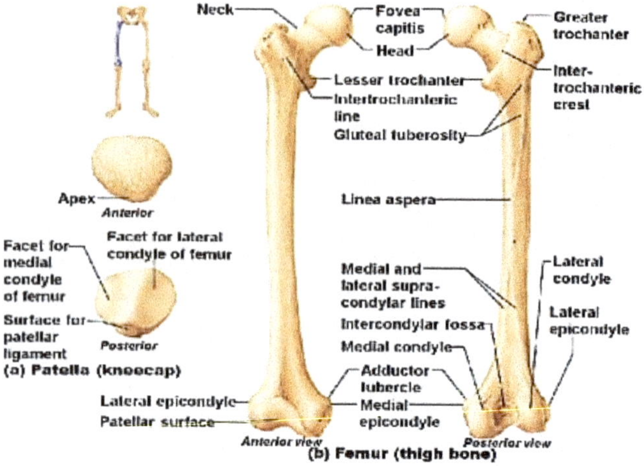

Fig. 44. Lower limbs.

2.4. Organization of skeletal muscle:

Skeletal muscle is a highly organized tissue that plays a crucial role in movement, posture, and overall body function.

Structural organization of skeletal muscle:

A. Muscle fiber (Muscle cell):

Description: Skeletal muscle fibers are long, cylindrical cells that can be several centimeters in length, each muscle fiber is a single cell with multiple nuclei, making it multinucleated.

Components are:

a. Sarcolemma: The plasma membrane of the muscle fiber.

b. Sarcoplasm: The cytoplasm of the muscle fiber, containing organelles such as mitochondria and myofibrils.

c. Myofibrils: Rod-like structures within the muscle fiber, composed of repeating units called sarcomeres.

d. Sarcomeres: The functional units of muscle contraction, made up of actin (thin filaments) and myosin (thick filaments) arranged in a specific pattern to create striations (striped appearance).

B. Fascicle:

Description: A fascicle is a bundle of muscle fibers. Several fascicles together form a whole muscle.

Connective tissue covering:

Perimysium: A layer of connective tissue that surrounds each fascicle, providing support and carrying blood vessels and nerves.

C. Whole muscle:
Description: The entire muscle is composed of multiple fascicles grouped together.
Connective tissue coverings: a. Epimysium: A dense layer of connective tissue that surrounds the entire muscle, protecting it and helping to transmit the force generated by muscle contraction to the tendons and bones.
b. Tendons: Strong, fibrous connective tissue that connects muscles to bones, they are continuous with the epimysium and periosteum (outer layer of bone).

Hierarchy of Muscle Organization:
a. Muscle Fiber: The basic unit, containing myofibrils.
b. Fascicle: A bundle of muscle fibers.
c. Muscle: A collection of fascicles working together as a single unit.

Functional organization of skeletal muscle includes:
I. Motor units:
Description: A motor unit consists of a motor neuron and all the muscle fibers it innervates, when the motor neuron sends a signal, all the fibers in the unit contract simultaneously.
Function: Motor units allow for graded muscle responses, meaning the strength of muscle contraction can vary depending on the number of motor units activated.

II. Neuromuscular junction:
Description: The synapse or junction between a motor neuron and a muscle fiber.
Function: It is the site where the nerve impulse (action potential) is transmitted from the neuron to the muscle fiber, initiating muscle contraction.

III. Sliding filament theory:
Description: Muscle contraction occurs through the sliding of actin (thin) and myosin (thick) filaments within the sarcomere. Myosin heads attach to actin and pull them towards the center of the sarcomere, shortening the muscle.
Function: This process underlies muscle contraction and is driven by ATP and calcium ions.

2.5. Physiology of muscle contraction: The physiology of muscle contraction involves a complex process where a muscle fiber generates tension through a series of biochemical and biophysical events. Here's a detailed explanation of how muscle contraction occurs:

Steps in muscle contraction:

i. Neuromuscular junction and excitation:

a. Nerve impulse: A muscle contraction begins when a motor neuron sends an electrical signal (action potential) down its axon to the neuromuscular junction, the synapse between the neuron and the muscle fiber.

b. Release of Acetylcholine (ACh): At the neuromuscular junction, the arrival of the nerve impulse triggers the release of the neurotransmitter acetylcholine (ACh) from synaptic vesicles into the synaptic cleft.

c. Binding of ACh to Receptors: Acetylcholine binds to receptors on the sarcolemma (muscle fiber membrane), causing ion channels to open and sodium ions (Na^+) to rush into the muscle fiber.

d. Depolarization: The influx of Na^+ depolarizes the sarcolemma, creating an action potential that travels along the membrane and down into the muscle fiber via structures called T-tubules.

ii. Excitation-contraction coupling:

a. T-tubules and Sarcoplasmic Reticulum: The action potential travels down the T-tubules, which are invaginations of the sarcolemma, and reaches the sarcoplasmic reticulum (SR), a specialized endoplasmic reticulum that stores calcium ions (Ca^{2+}).

b. Release of Calcium Ions: The action potential triggers the SR to release Ca^{2+} into the sarcoplasm (cytoplasm of the muscle fiber).

c. Calcium Binding: Calcium ions bind to troponin, a regulatory protein associated with the thin filament (actin).

iii. Cross-bridge formation:

a. Troponin-Tropomyosin Complex: In a resting muscle, tropomyosin blocks the active sites on actin, preventing myosin heads from binding, when calcium binds to troponin, it causes a conformational change that moves tropomyosin away from these active sites.

b. Myosin-Actin Binding: With the active sites exposed, the myosin heads (part of the thick filament) bind to actin, forming a cross-bridge.

iv. Power stroke and energy release:

a. ADP and Phosphate release: The myosin head releases ADP and inorganic phosphate (Pi), which were products of ATP hydrolysis in the resting state.

b. Power stroke: The release of ADP and Pi causes the myosin head to pivot and pull the actin filament toward the center of the sarcomere, shortening the muscle fiber, this is known as the power stroke.

v. Detachment and reorganize:
a. Binding of ATP: A new ATP molecule binds to the myosin head, causing it to detach from the actin filament.
b. ATP hydrolysis: The myosin head hydrolyzes the ATP into ADP and Pi, providing the energy required to reorganize (reset) the myosin head into its high-energy position, ready for another cycle of contraction.

vi. Relaxation:
a. Cessation of nerve signal: When the nerve signal stops, acetylcholine is broken down by the enzyme acetylcholinesterase, closing the ion channels on the sarcolemma and halting the action potential.
b. Reuptake of calcium: Calcium ions are actively transported back into the sarcoplasmic reticulum, decreasing their concentration in the sarcoplasm.
c. Tropomyosin blockage: As calcium levels drop, troponin returns to its original shape, causing tropomyosin to once again cover the active sites on actin. This prevents further cross-bridge formation, and the muscle fiber relaxes.

2.6. Neuromuscular junction:

The neuromuscular junction is a specialized synapse where a motor neuron communicates with a skeletal muscle fiber to initiate muscle contraction, it is crucial for translating neural signals into physical movement.

Structure of the neuromuscular junction:
i. Motor neuron:
a. Axon terminal: The end of the motor neuron that approaches the muscle fiber, it contains synaptic vesicles filled with the neurotransmitter acetylcholine (ACh).
b. Synaptic vesicles: Membrane-bound sacs within the axon terminal that store and release acetylcholine into the synaptic cleft upon stimulation.

ii. Synaptic cleft:
Description: A small gap between the axon terminal of the motor neuron and the muscle fiber's sarcolemma (plasma membrane).
Function: The synaptic cleft allows the diffusion of acetylcholine from the neuron to the muscle fiber.

iii. Motor end plate:
Description: The specialized region of the muscle fiber's sarcolemma directly across from the axon terminal. It contains junctional folds to increase surface area.
Acetylcholine receptors: Nicotinic receptors located on the motor end plate that bind acetylcholine and are responsible for initiating the muscle action potential.

Function of the neuromuscular junction:
a. Nerve impulse arrival: An action potential travels down the motor neuron to the axon terminal, triggering the opening of voltage-gated calcium channels.
b. Release of Acetylcholine: The influx of calcium ions into the axon terminal causes synaptic vesicles to fuse with the presynaptic membrane, releasing acetylcholine into the synaptic cleft by exocytosis.
c. Acetylcholine binding: Acetylcholine diffuses across the synaptic cleft and binds to acetylcholine receptors on the motor end plate of the muscle fiber.
d. Muscle action potential: Binding of acetylcholine to its receptors opens ion channels, allowing sodium ions (Na^+) to enter the muscle fiber. this depolarizes the sarcolemma, creating an action potential that spreads across the muscle fiber, initiating contraction.
e. Acetylcholine breakdown: The enzyme acetylcholinesterase, present in the synaptic cleft, rapidly breaks down acetylcholine into acetic acid and choline. This stops the signal, allowing the muscle fiber to relax.
f. Recycling of components: Choline is taken back up by the neuron's axon terminal for reuse in synthesizing new acetylcholine molecules.

Unit – 2.

Chapter 3.

Joints

Joints, or articulations, are anatomical structures that join bones in the body, enabling movement and providing mechanical support. They can be categorized according to their structure and function.

A. Classification of connections may be done based on their structure known as "structural classification":

I. Connective tissue joints:
Description: The bones are connected by dense fibrous tissue, eliminating the need for a joint cavity.
Types of connective tissue joints are:
a. Sutures in the skull are classified as immovable joints, specifically known as synarthrosis.
b. Syndesmoses refer to the connection of bones by ligaments, which permits limited mobility known as amphiarthrosis, an example of this is the distal tibiofibular joint.
c. Gomphoses are synarthroses, joints characterized by immovable peg-in-socket connections, such as the connection between the teeth and the jaw.

II. Cartilaginous joints:
Description: Bones are connected by cartilage, with no joint cavity.
Types of cartilaginous joints are:
Synchondroses: Bones united by hyaline cartilage, usually immovable (synarthrosis), e.g., the epiphyseal plates in growing bones.
Symphyses: Bones united by fibrocartilage, allowing limited movement (amphiarthrosis), e.g., the intervertebral discs and pubic symphysis.

III. Synovial Joints:
Description: Bones are separated by a fluid-filled joint cavity, allowing free movement (diarthrosis).
The following parts are:
a. Articular cartilage: Hyaline cartilage that covers the ends of bones, reducing friction.

b. Joint cavity: A space containing synovial fluid, which lubricates the joint.
c. Articular Capsule: A two-layered capsule surrounding the joint, with an outer fibrous layer and an inner synovial membrane.
d. Synovial Fluid: A lubricating fluid secreted by the synovial membrane.
e. Ligaments: Bands of dense connective tissue that reinforce the joint.
f. Bursae and Tendon Sheaths: Fluid-filled sacs and tubular structures that reduce friction between tendons and bones or skin.

B. "Functional classification":
a. Synarthroses: immovable joints, e.g., skull sutures. Amphiarthrosis: Easily movable joints, such as intervertebral discs.
b. Diarthroses: freely mobile joints, e.g., most synovial joints, such as the shoulder, hip, and knee.

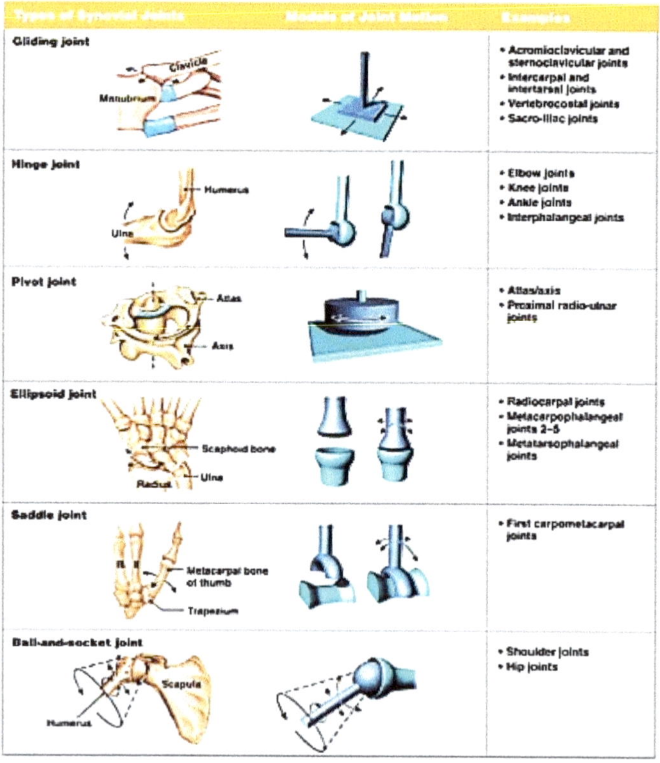

Fig. 45. Joints.

Types of synovial joints:
a. Planar joints, also known as gliding joints or sliding joints:
Movement: Gliding or gliding movements, such as the intercarpal joints of the wrist

b. Hinge joints, or joints of joints, move through flexion and extension, similar to a door hinge, such as the elbow and knee joints.

c. Pivot joints or swivel joints Movement: Rotation around one axis, e.g., atlantoaxial joint (between the first and second cervical vertebrae).

d. Condyloid (ellipsoid) joints
Movement includes flexion, extension, abduction, adduction, and circumduction, for example, in the wrist.

e. Saddle joints
Movement: Similar to condyloid joints but with a greater range of motion, e.g., the carpometacarpal joint of the thumb.

f. Ball and socket joints
Movement: Most freely movable joints are shoulder and hip joints, allow flexion, extension, abduction, adduction, rotation, and circumduction.

3.1. The structural and functional classification of joints are:
Each classification helps to understand how joints connect bones and their movement capabilities.
I. Structural classification:
A structural classification categorizes joints based on the material connecting the bones and the presence or absence of a joint cavity.
A. Fibrous joints: Dense fibrous tissue connects the bones; there is no joint cavity.
The following types are:
a. Sutures:
Characteristics: The skull contains immovable joints; a thin layer of connective tissue firmly connects the bones; an example of this is the sagittal suture between the parietal bones.
b. Syndesmosis:
Characteristics: Connected by a ligament or interosseous membrane, allowing limited movement; an example is the distal tibiofibular joint.

c. Gomphoses:
characteristics: The joints, such as the connection between the tooth and the alveolar cavity, are where the tooth fits into the bony socket of the jaw.

B. Cartilaginous joints: Bones are connected by cartilage. There is no joint cavity.
The following types are:
a. Synchondrosis:
Hyaline cartilage, often immobile, connects bones; an example of this is the epiphyseal plates in growing bones.
b. Symphyses:
Fibrous cartilage connects bones, allowing limited movement; examples include intervertebral discs and pubic symphysis.

C. Synovial joints: A fluid-filled joint cavity separates the bones, allowing for free movement.
The following parts are:
a. Articular cartilage is the tissue that covers the ends of bones.
b. Joint cavity: filled with synovial fluid.
c. Joint capsule: the outer fibrous layer and inner synovial membrane that surround the joint.
d. Synovial fluid: Lubricates the joint.
e. Ligaments: strengthening the joint.
f. Bursae and tendon sheaths: Lower friction.

II. Functional classification:
Functional classification categorizes joints based on the degree of movement allowed.
a. Synarthroses: Immovable joints or fixed connections; examples are stitches in the skull, gomphoses between the teeth and jaw, synchondroses in the epiphyseal plates.

b. Amphiarthrosis: Easily movable joints; examples are symphyses such as intervertebral discs and pubic symphysis, syndesmoses such as the distal tibiofibular joint.

c. Diarthrosis: Freely movable joints.
The following types are:
i. Hinge joints: These joints, like the elbow and knee, allow for flexion and extension.
ii. Pivot (swivel) joints: These joints, such as the atlantoaxial joint, enable rotational movement.

iii. Condyloid joints: These joints, such as the wrist joint, allow movement in two planes.
iv. Saddle joints: These joints allow for a variety of movements, including those that are opposed, such as the thumb joint.
v. Ball joints: Enable movement in multiple axes (e.g., shoulder and hip joints).

3.2. Types of joint movements and their articulation:
There are several types of joint movements and their corresponding articulations are:
I. Flexion and extension bending:
a. Flexion: This action reduces the angle between two body parts and brings them closer together, such as when an elbow or knee is bent.
b. Extension: This process increases the angle between two body parts and straightens them; an example of this would be straightening an arm or leg after flexion.

Flexion and extension articulations are:
a. Hinge joints, such as the elbow and knee, allow movement primarily in one plane.
b. Ball-and-socket joints: For example, the shoulder and hip joints allow flexion and extension in multiple planes.

II. Abduction and adduction:
Abduction is the movement of a body part away from the center line of the body, such as raising an arm or leg to the side.
b. Adduction: The movement of a body part towards the midline of the body, such as returning your arm or leg to the center of your body.

Abduction and adduction articulations are:
a. Ball-and-socket joints, similar to the shoulder and hip, allow abduction and adduction.
b. Saddle joints: The thumb joint, for instance, enables a range of motion that includes abduction and adduction.

III. Rotation:
The movement of a body part around its own axis is described as follows:
Types: a. Medial rotation: rotation toward the midline of the body.
b. Lateral rotation refers to a rotation that is directed away from the midline of the body, such as turning your head to look over your shoulder.

Rotation articulations:

a. Pivot joints: One such example is the atlantoaxial joint in the neck, which facilitates rotational movement.
b. Ball-and-socket joints, such as the shoulder and hip joints, which also allow for rotation.

IV. Circumduction:
Description: A circular movement of a part of the body creates a cone-shaped movement; an example of this would be moving the arm in a circular motion to perform a windmill motion.

Circumduction articulations:
a. Ball-and-socket joints, such as the shoulder and hip joints, allow for circumduction due to their wide range of motion.
b. Condyloid joints: For instance, a wrist capable of varying degrees of circumduction.

V. Supination and pronation:
a. Supination: rotation of the forearm so that the palm faces upwards or forwards; example: holding a bowl of soup.
b. Pronation: rotation of the forearm so that the palm faces down or back; example: turning the hand and placing it on the table, palm down.

Supination and pronation articulations:
a. Pivot joints: The proximal radioulnar joint, for instance, facilitates the pronation and supination of the forearm.

VI. Elevation and depression:
a. Elevation refers to the final lift of a body part, such as shrugging.
b. Depression: The act of lowering a body part inferiorly; for instance, lowering the shoulders after shrugging.

Elevation and depression articulation:
a. Saddle joints, such as the sternoclavicular joint, allow for elevation and depression.
b. Ball joints, like the shoulder, are capable of performing these movements to a certain degree.

VII. Opposition and reposition:
a. Opposition: The movement of the thumb and little finger towards each other, exemplified by a pinching motion.
b. Repositioning involves moving the thumb and little finger away from each other, such as returning them to their initial positions.

Opposition and reposition articulation:
Saddle joints, like the carpometacarpal joint of the thumb, facilitate opposition and repositioning.

Related questions from unit 2

1. Differentiate between skeletal and smooth muscle.
2. Describe in brief about the dermis layer of skin.
3. Describe in brief about the epidermal layer of the skin.
4. Describe in brief about the thermo-regulation in human body.
5. Describe in brief about sweat gland.
6. Describe the process of healing of fractures.
7. Describe the bones present in the human skull.
8. Describe the bones present in the vertebral column.
9. Describe in brief about thoracic cage.
10. Describe in brief about the appendicular skeleton.
11. Describe in brief about the structure and function of synovial joint.
12. Explain the structure and function of skin.
13. Briefly classify the types of bones present in human body.
14. Write in detail about wound healing?
15. Explain in detail about axial skeletal system.
16. Explain the organization of skeletal muscle.
17. Explain the joint moments and its articulations.
18. Explain in detail about physiology of muscle contraction
19. Explain in detail about the neuromuscular junction.
20. Explain in detail about the healing of fractures.

Unit – 3.

Topic	Page no.
Chapter 1: Body fluids and blood	91
1.1. Body fluids	91 – 93
1.2. Composition and functions of blood	93 – 95
1.3. Haematopoiesis	95
1.4. Hemoglobin formation	95 – 96
1.5. Anemia	96
1.6. Mechanisms of coagulation, or blood clotting	97 – 98
1.7. Blood groups	98 – 99
1.8. Rh factors	99 – 100
1.9. Transfusion	100
1.10. Transfusion significance and blood disorders	100 – 101
1.11. Reticulo-endothelial system	101 – 102

Topic	Page no.
Chapter 2: Lymphatic system	103
2.1. Lymphatic organs and tissues	104 – 105
2.2. Lymphatic vessels	105 – 106
2.3. Lymph circulation	106 – 107
2.4. Functions of lymphatic system	107

Related questions from unit 3	108

Unit – 3.

Chapter 1.

Body fluids and blood

1.1. Body fluids: Those are the liquid components found in various parts of the human body, including blood, interstitial fluid, and intracellular fluid. Blood is a key type of body fluid with specific functions and properties:

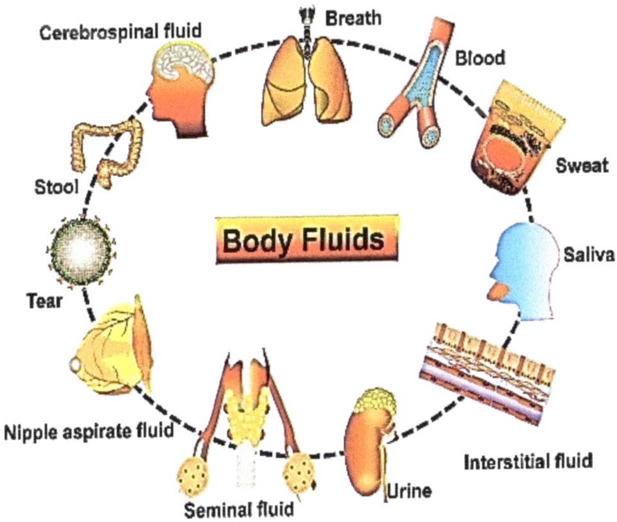

Fig. 46. Body Fluids.

I. Types of body fluids:

a. Intracellular fluid (ICF): Fluid found inside cells.
Volume: Makes up about 60% of total body fluid volume.

Function: Provides a medium for cellular processes and helps maintain cell shape and function.

b. Extracellular fluid (ECF): This fluid is located outside cells and can be further divided into different compartments.

Subdivision of extracellular fluids:
i. Interstitial fluid: Fluid that surrounds cells and fills the spaces between them.
Function: Acts as a medium for the exchange of nutrients, gases and waste products between blood and cells.
ii. Plasma: The liquid component of blood that circulates in the blood vessels.
Function: Transports cells, nutrients, hormones and waste products throughout the body.
iii. Transcellular fluid: Description: Specialized fluids contained in specific compartments (e.g. cerebrospinal fluid, synovial fluid).
Function: Performs various specific roles depending on its location, such as cushioning the brain or lubricating the joints.

c. Body fluid balance: Maintaining the correct volume and composition of body fluids.
Regulation: Mechanisms such as thirst, hormonal regulation (e.g., antidiuretic hormone, aldosterone), and kidney function are controlled.

II. Blood:
a. Composition of plasma: It is the liquid component of blood, accounting for about 55% of its volume, the components are:
i. Water: Approximately 90% of plasma.
ii. Electrolytes: Sodium, potassium, calcium, chloride, bicarbonate.
iii. Proteins: Albumin (maintains osmotic pressure), globulins (immune response), fibrinogen (blood clotting).
iv. Nutrients and waste products: Glucose, amino acids, urea, hormones.
v. Formed elements: The cellular components of blood that make up about 45% of its volume.
vi. Red blood cells (erythrocytes): Description: Biconcave discs that transport oxygen from the lungs to the tissues and carbon dioxide from the tissues to the lungs.

b. Functions: Transport of oxygen, removal of carbon dioxide, its lifespan about 120 days and white blood cells (i.e., leukocytes) these are cells that are involved in immune responses and infection defence.

c. Types: Neutrophils, lymphocytes, monocytes, eosinophils, basophils.

Functions: Immunity, destruction of pathogens.

d. Platelets (thrombocytes): Description: Small cell fragments involved in blood clotting.

Functions of blood:
i. The process involves the formation of blood clots and the healing of wounds. (Duration: About 7-10 days.)
ii. Blood function Transportation: Oxygen and carbon dioxide transferred between the lungs and tissues.
iii. Nutrients and wastes: Transferred from the digestive system to the cells and waste products to the kidneys.
iv. Hormones: Transported from endocrine glands to target organs.
v. Body temperature: Blood distributes heat to help regulate temperature.
vi. pH balance: Blood buffers keep the pH within a narrow range.
vii. Fluid balance: This ensures that tissues and blood vessels maintain the proper fluid levels.
viii. Protection: Immune function: White blood cells and antibodies protect against pathogens.
ix. Clotting: Platelets and clotting factors prevent excessive bleeding from injuries.

III. Blood circulation:
a. systemic circulation: The aorta transports blood from the left side of the heart to the rest of the body, and the veins return the blood to the right side of the heart.
b. Pulmonary Circulation: The right side of the heart pumps blood to the lungs for oxygenation, after which it returns to the left side of the heart.

1.2. Blood composition and functions:
Blood is a vital fluid in the body that performs several critical functions required for survival. It consists of fluid and cellular components, each of which has a specific role:
I. Blood composition: Blood consists of two main components: plasma and formed elements.
A. Plasma: A liquid component of blood that makes up about 55% of its total volume.
Components:
a. Water: Approximately 90% plasma; serves as a solvent and medium for the transport of substances.

b. Electrolytes: These include sodium, potassium, calcium, chloride, bicarbonate and others; they help maintain osmotic balance,
c. pH balance and the proper functioning of cells and tissues.
d. Proteins:
i. Albumin, maintains osmotic pressure, prevents fluid loss from blood vessels to tissues.
ii. Globulins: This category includes antibodies, also known as immunoglobulins, which participate in immune reactions.
iii. Fibrinogen: When a clot forms, it transforms into fibrin, which is essential for blood clotting.
iv. Nutrients: Includes glucose, amino acids, lipids and vitamins; supplies cells with energy and building blocks. v. Wastes: Such as urea, creatinine and bilirubin; transported to excretory organs for elimination.
vi. Hormones: Target organs receive a variety of hormones that regulate physiological processes.

B. Formed elements: The cellular components of blood make up about 45% of its total volume, the components are:
i. Red blood cell (Erythrocytes): It is biconcave disc-shaped cells without a nucleus make up red blood cells, also known as erythrocytes.
Function:
a. Transporting oxygen from the lungs to the tissues and carbon dioxide from the tissues to the lungs.
b. Shelf life: Approximately 120 days.

ii. White blood cells, also known as leukocytes, are cells involved in the immune response, they have a nucleus and come in various types:
i. Neutrophils: Play a role in the phagocytosis of pathogens and debris.
ii. Lymphocytes: This includes T cells and B cells that are involved in adaptive immunity.
iii. Monocytes: Differentiate into macrophages that phagocytose pathogens and dead cells.
iv. Eosinophils: Fight parasitic infections and modulate allergic reactions.
v. Basophils: Release histamine and other chemicals during allergic reactions.
Function: Protects the body from infection and foreign substances.
vi. Platelets (thrombocytes): Small cell fragments derived from megakaryocytes.
Functions: They play a key role in blood clotting by clumping together at sites of injury to form clots. Duration: About 7-10 days.

II. Blood function: Blood carries out a number of fundamental tasks, such as:

A. Transportation:
i. Oxygen: Transports oxygen from the lungs to the tissues and cells.
ii. Carbon Dioxide: This gas transports carbon dioxide from the tissues to the lungs for exhalation.
iii. Nutrients: Delivers nutrients absorbed from the digestive tract to cells.
iv. Waste: Transports waste products to the kidneys, liver and other organs for excretion.
v. Hormones: Carries hormones from endocrine glands to target organs.

B. Regulations:
i. Body Temperature: Helps regulate body temperature by distributing and dispersing heat.
ii. pH balance: Maintains the acid-base balance in the blood by means of buffering systems that contain primarily bicarbonate.
iii. Fluid balance: Regulates fluid volume in blood and tissues, affects blood pressure and tissue hydration.

C. Protection:
i. Immune response: White blood cells and antibodies protect the body from infections, pathogens and foreign substances.
ii. Clotting: Platelets and clotting factors work together to prevent excessive bleeding and facilitate wound healing.

1.3. Haematopoiesis:
Haematopoiesis is the process by which blood cells are formed, this complex process occurs primarily in the bone marrow and involves the differentiation of stem cells into different types of blood cells, including red blood cells (erythrocytes), white blood cells (leukocytes), and platelets (platelets).
There are two main types of hemopoiesis:
a. Myeloid hemopoiesis: Occurs in the bone marrow and is responsible for the production of red blood cells, platelets, and most types of white blood cells (except lymphocytes).
b. Lymphoid hemopoiesis: Occurs in the lymphatic system and is responsible for the production of lymphocytes, a type of white blood cell involved in the immune response.
The hematopoietic process is regulated by various growth factors and cytokines that stimulate the proliferation and differentiation of hematopoietic stem cells, these stem cells are multipotent, meaning they have the ability to develop into different types of blood cells depending on the signals they receive.

1.4. Haemoglobin formation: Haemoglobin formation, or haemoglobin synthesis, occurs primarily in the bone marrow and involves several key steps:

i. Hematopoietic stem cells: The process begins with hematopoietic stem cells in the bone marrow that differentiate into erythroid progenitor cells.

ii. Erythropoiesis: These progenitor cells go through a series of stages to become mature red blood cells (erythrocytes); during this process, they lose their nucleus and organelles.

iii. Synthesis of globin chains: Haemoglobin is a protein composed of four polypeptide chains, typically two alpha (α) and two beta (β) chains in adults (HbA), the synthesis of these chains occurs in the ribosomes of developing erythrocytes, the genes for the globin chains are located on different chromosomes (alpha chains on chromosome 16 and beta chains on chromosome 11).

iv. Heme Production: Heme, the iron-containing component of haemoglobin, is synthesized in the mitochondria and cytoplasm of erythroid cells. The process involves several steps, starting with a porphyrin precursor molecule that is converted to heme by a series of enzymatic reactions.

v. Assembly of Haemoglobin: Once the globin chains and heme groups are formed, they combine to form haemoglobin, each molecule of haemoglobin can bind to four molecules of oxygen, allowing red blood cells to transport oxygen throughout the body.

vi. Release into circulation: Once the mature red blood cells, now containing haemoglobin, are released into the bloodstream where they perform their function of transporting oxygen.

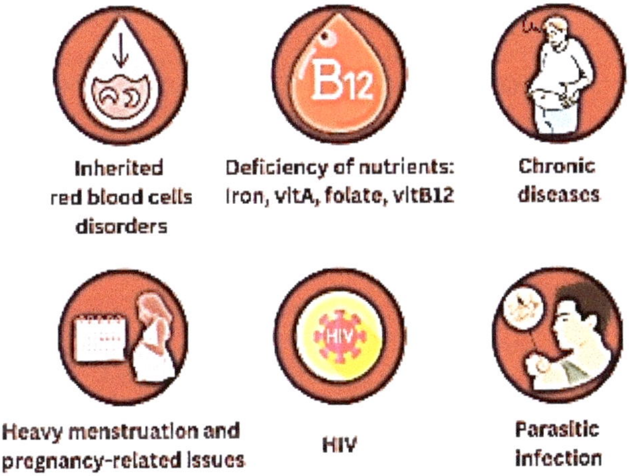

Fig. 47. Factors causing anaemia.

1.5. Anaemia: Anaemia is a condition characterized by a lack of red blood cells or haemoglobin in the blood, which can lead to reduced oxygen transport to body tissues, there are several types and causes of anaemia, including:

a. Iron deficiency anaemia: The most common type, caused by a lack of iron, which is necessary for the formation of haemoglobin, this can be caused by insufficient food intake, blood loss (e.g., during menstruation or gastrointestinal bleeding) or increased need (e.g., during pregnancy).

b. Vitamin deficiency anaemia: This can occur due to a lack of certain vitamins, especially vitamin B12 and folic acid, which are essential for the formation of red blood cells.

c. Anaemia of chronic disease: Conditions such as chronic kidney disease, cancer, or inflammatory diseases can interfere with the production of red blood cells.

d. Aplastic anaemia: A rare but serious condition in which the bone marrow fails to produce enough red blood cells, often due to autoimmune diseases, exposure to toxic substances, or certain medications.

e. Haemolytic anaemia: This occurs when red blood cells are destroyed faster than they can be produced, causes may include autoimmune disorders, infections, or certain hereditary conditions.

Symptoms of anaemia can vary, but often include fatigue, weakness, pale skin, shortness of breath, and dizziness.

Diagnosis usually involves blood tests to measure haemoglobin levels and assess the number of red blood cells.
Treatment depends on the underlying cause and may include dietary changes, supplements (such as iron or vitamins), medications, or procedures to address the underlying cause of the anaemia. coagulation

1.6. Mechanisms of coagulation, or blood clotting:
It is a complex process that prevents excessive bleeding when a vessel is injured, it involves a series of steps that can generally be divided into three main phases: vasospasm, platelet plug formation, and the coagulation cascade.
i. Vascular spasm: Immediate response when a blood vessel is injured, the smooth muscle in the vessel wall contracts, leading to vasoconstriction, this reduces blood flow to the area and minimizes blood loss.

ii. Plate plug formation: It goes through 3 process:
a. Platelets adherence to exposed collagen fibers in the damaged vessel wall, this is facilitated by Von Willebrand factor (VWF), which acts as a bridge between platelets and collagen.
b. Platelet activation: Once attached, platelets become activated and change shape, releasing chemical signals (such as ADP, thromboxane-A2, and serotonin) that attract more platelets to the site of injury.
c. Platelet Aggregation: Collected platelets stick together to form a temporary "platelet plug" that covers the injury.

iii. Coagulation cascade: This phase involves a series of enzymatic reactions that lead to the conversion of fibrinogen (a soluble plasma protein) to fibrin (an insoluble protein), which stabilizes the platelet plug.
a. Intrinsic pathway: Activated by damage to a blood vessel and involves several coagulation factors (factors XII, XI, IX, and VIII), this pathway is slower and is often triggered by internal damage.
b. Extrinsic pathway: This pathway is triggered by external trauma to a blood vessel and is initiated by tissue factor (TF) released from damaged tissues and includes factor VII, it is faster than the internal route.
c. Common pathway: Both pathways converge at factor X, resulting in the conversion of prothrombin (factor II) to thrombin (factor IIa), thrombin then converts fibrinogen to fibrin, which forms a meshwork that solidifies the platelet plug.

iv. Clot retraction and repair:

a. Clot retraction: Platelets contract and pull the edges of the wound closer together, helping tissue repair.
b. Fibrinolysis: Once the vessel is healed, the clot is removed by a process called fibrinolysis, where plasminogen is converted to plasmin, which breaks down the fibrin and dissolves the clot.

Blood Type	Donate Blood To	Receive Blood From
A+	A+ AB+	A+ A- O+ O-
O+	O+ A+ B+ AB+	O+ O-
B+	B+ AB+	B+ B- O+ O-
AB+	AB+	Everyone
A-	A+ A- AB+ AB-	A- O-
O-	Everyone	O-
B-	B+ B- AB+ AB-	B- O-
AB-	AB+ AB-	AB- A- B- O-

Table No. 01. Blood group types

1.7. Blood groups:
Blood groups are a system used to classify blood based on the presence or absence of specific antigens on the surface of red blood cells, the most well-known blood group systems are the ABO and Rh systems.
a. ABO blood group system: The ABO system classifies blood into four main groups:
i. Type A: It has A antigens on the surface of red blood cells and B antibodies in the plasma.
ii. Type B: Contains B antigens on the surface of red blood cells and A antibodies in the plasma.
iii. Type AB: It has both A and B antigens on the surface of red blood cells and no A or B antibodies in the plasma, this is known as a universal recipient.
iv. Type O: Has neither A nor B antigens on the surface of red blood cells, but has both A and B antibodies in the plasma, this is known as a universal donor.

Rh blood group system: The Rh system is based on the presence or absence of the Rh factor (also known as the D antigen): Rh-positive

(Rh+): If the Rh factor is present on red blood cells. Rh-negative (Rh-): If the Rh factor is missing.
Importance of blood groups: Blood grouping is important for several reasons:
a. Transfusion: Ensures compatibility of donor and recipient blood to avoid adverse reactions.
b. Pregnancy: Helps manage Rh incompatibility between mother and foetus.
c. Organ transplantation: Helps find donors and recipients to reduce the risk of rejection.
d. Blood group testing: Blood typing is usually done using a simple blood test where the sample is mixed with specific antibodies to determine the presence of A, B and Rh antigens.

1.8. Rh factors:
The Rh factor, also known as the Rhesus factor, is a protein that can be present on the surface of red blood cells, it is one of the key components in determining a person's blood group along with the ABO blood group system.

Types of Rh factor:
a. Rh positive (Rh+): If your blood has the Rh protein, you are considered Rh positive.
b. Rh negative (Rh-): If your blood lacks the Rh protein, you are considered Rh negative.
The importance of the Rh factor Pregnancy: Rh incompatibility can occur when a Rh-negative mother carries a Rh-positive baby, this can lead to haemolytic disease of the new-born (HDN), where the mother's immune system attacks the baby's red blood cells.

1.9. Blood transfusion:
In order to avoid adverse reactions, it is very important that the blood transfusion corresponds to the Rh factor.
i. Rh-negative person should receive Rh-negative blood to avoid complications.
ii. Organ transplants: Rh matching may also be important in organ transplants to reduce the risk of rejection. Rh factor testing Rh factor is typically determined during blood typing, which involves mixing a blood sample with specific antibodies that react to the Rh protein.
iii. Transfusion: Blood transfusions involve the transfer of blood or blood components from one person (the donor) to another (the recipient), especially as they relate to the Rh factor:

The importance of the Rh factor in transfusions are:
i. Compatibility: It is important to match the Rh factor of the donor and recipient to avoid adverse reactions. For example, an Rh-negative person should ideally receive Rh-negative blood to avoid complications.
ii. Rh incompatibility: If a Rh-negative person receives Rh-positive blood, their immune system may produce antibodies against the Rh factor, leading to a potentially serious reaction.
iii. Universal donor and recipient:
Universal donor: Type O negative blood is considered a universal donor because it lacks A, B, and Rh antigens, making it safe for most recipients.
Universal Recipient: Type AB positive blood is considered a universal recipient because it has all the antigens and can accept any blood type.

Types of blood components:
a. Whole blood: Contains all the components of blood.
i. Red blood cells (RBCs): Transfusions are often given to treat anaemia or blood loss.
ii. Platelets: Used in patients with low platelet counts.
iii. Plasma: The liquid part of blood, given for various conditions, testing before transfusion prior to transfusion, blood grouping and cross-checking are performed to ensure donor and recipient blood compatibility.

1.10. Transfusion significance and blood disorders:
Blood plays a vital role in the body and its importance can be understood through its various functions and components.
a. Significance of blood Transport: Blood transports oxygen from the lungs to the body's tissues and carbon dioxide from the tissues back to the lungs, it also transports nutrients from the digestive tract and hormones from the endocrine glands to various parts of the body.
b. Regulation:
i. Blood helps regulate body temperature, pH levels and fluid balance.
ii. it maintains homeostasis by adjusting heat distribution and electrolyte concentration.
iii. Protection: Blood contains white blood cells and antibodies, which are essential for the immune response and help defend the body against infections and foreign invaders.
iv. Platelets and clotting factors in the blood are key to healing wounds and preventing excessive bleeding.
v. Blood Clotting: Blood has the ability to clot, which is vital to stop bleeding when an injury occurs.

Common blood disorders:

a. Anaemia: A condition characterized by a lack of red blood cells or haemoglobin, resulting in reduced oxygen transport, it can have a variety of causes, including nutritional deficiencies (iron, vitamin B12, folate), chronic disease, or bone marrow disorders.

b. Leukemia: A type of cancer that affects the blood and bone marrow, leading to an overproduction of abnormal white blood cells, this can disrupt the normal formation and function of blood cells.

c. Haemophilia: A genetic disorder that impairs the blood's ability to clot, leading to excessive bleeding, this is often due to a lack of specific triggering factors.

d. Thrombocytopenia: A condition characterized by low platelet counts that can lead to increased bleeding and bruising, it can be caused by a number of factors, including bone marrow disorders, autoimmune diseases, or certain medications.

e. Sickle cell disease: A genetic disorder in which red blood cells become misshapen (sickle-shaped), leading to blocked blood vessels, pain, and an increased risk of infection.

f. Polycythaemia Vera: A rare blood disorder in which the bone marrow produces too many red blood cells, leading to increased blood viscosity and a higher risk of thrombosis.

g. Blood clots (thrombosis): Abnormal clotting can lead to conditions such as deep vein thrombosis (DVT) or pulmonary embolism (PE), which can be life-threatening.

1.11. Reticular Endothelial System:

The reticuloendothelial system (RES), now more commonly referred to as the mononuclear phagocytic system (MPS), is a network of cells and tissues that play a key role in the immune response and the removal of pathogens, dead cells, and other debris in bloodstream.

a. RES/MPS Folders Monocytes and macrophages: Monocytes are white blood cells that circulate in the bloodstream and can differentiate into macrophages when migrating into tissues, macrophages are essential for phagocytosis, the process of engulfing and digesting cellular debris and pathogens.

b. Dendritic cells: These cells are important for antigen presentation and play a key role in the initiation of the adaptive immune response.

c. Kupffer cells: Located in the liver, Kupffer cells are specialized macrophages that help filter the blood and remove pathogens and dead cells.

d. Spleen and lymph nodes: These organs contain a variety of immune cells, including macrophages and dendritic cells, which help filter blood and lymph.

e. Bone Marrow: A production site for monocytes and other blood cells, contributing to the overall function of the RES.
f. RES/MPS function Phagocytosis: The primary function of the RES is to engulf and digest pathogens, dead cells, and other debris.
g. Immune surveillance: RES cells constantly monitor the body for signs of infection or injury.
h. Antigen: Dendritic cells and macrophages present antigens to T cells, triggering an adaptive immune response.
i. Cytokine production: These cells produce various cytokines that help regulate immune responses and inflammation.
Clinical significance Disorders of RES can lead to a number of health problems, including infections, autoimmune diseases, and cancer. Understanding RES is key to developing treatments for these conditions.

Unit – 3.

Chapter 2.

Lymphatic systems

The lymphatic system is a key part of the immune system and plays a vital role in maintaining fluid balance in the body.

The lymphatic system's components include:

a. Lymphatic vessels: These are a network of vessels that transport lymph, a clear fluid that contains immune cells, proteins, and waste products. Lymphatic vessels are similar to veins but have thinner walls and more valves.

b. Lymph: This is the fluid that circulates through the lymphatic system. Lymphatic vessels collect the interstitial fluid that leaks from blood vessels into tissues.

c. Lymph nodes: These are small bean-shaped structures that filter lymph and store immune cells, such as lymphocytes and macrophages. They are important in the immune response because they capture pathogens and facilitate their destruction.

d. Spleen: The spleen filters the blood, removes old or damaged red blood cells, and helps produce lymphocytes. It also aids the immune system by responding to blood-borne pathogens.

e. Thymus: This is where T lymphocytes (T cells) mature. The thymus is especially important during childhood and adolescence.

f. Tonsils and adenoids: These are lymphoid tissues located in the throat that help protect against pathogens entering the mouth and nose.

The lymphatic system functions are:

i. The lymphatic system maintains fluid balance by returning excess interstitial fluid to the bloodstream, preventing edema (swelling).

ii. The immune response plays a crucial role in the immune system by transporting lymphocytes and other immune cells throughout the body. When pathogens are detected, lymph nodes filter lymph and initiate immune responses.

iii. The lymphatic system absorbs fats and fat-soluble vitamins from the digestive system through specialized lymphatic vessels called lacteals located in the small intestine.

iv. Waste Removal: Helps to eliminate waste products and cellular debris from tissues.

Clinical significance:

Disorders of the lymphatic system can lead to a number of health problems, including:

a. Lymphedema: swelling due to accumulation of lymphatic fluid, often caused by damage to lymph vessels or nodes, infections can occur, such as lymphangitis (inflammation of the lymph vessels) or lymphadenitis (inflammation of the lymph nodes).

b. Cancer: Lymphatic spread is a common pathway for cancer metastasis.

2.1. Lymphatic organs and tissues:

The lymphatic system is a network of organs, tissues, and vessels that play a vital role in our immune system function and overall health.

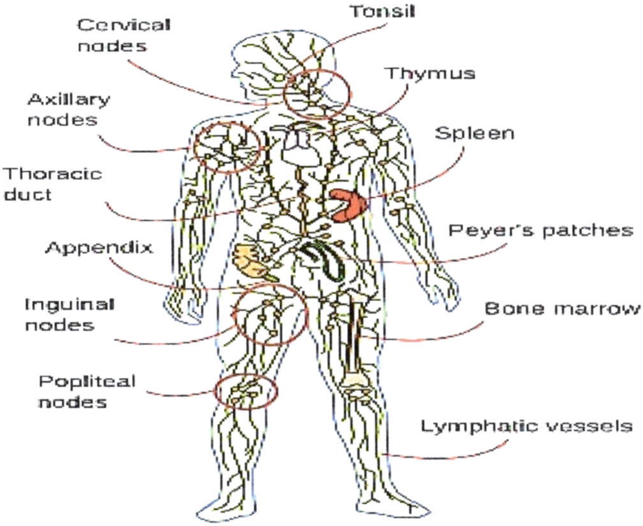

Fig. 48. Lymphatic organs.

Lymphatic organs:

i. Primary lymphatic organs: The bone marrow produces lymphocytes (B cells and T cells) and other immune cells, e.g., thymus: located behind the sternum, T cells mature and develop here.

ii. Secondary lymphatic organs: Lymph nodes (almost around 600-700 in the body): filter lymphatic fluids, trap pathogens, and activate immune responses, e.g., a. Cervical lymph nodes (neck), b. Axillary lymph nodes (armpit), c. Inguinal lymph nodes (groins).

iii. Spleens filter blood, store red blood cells, and detect and remove pathogens.

iv. Tonsils: masses of lymphoid tissue in the throat that help filter out pathogens.

v. Adenoids: lymphoid tissue at the back of the nasal passages that helps filter out pathogens.

vi. Peyer's patches: small masses of lymphoid tissue in the small intestine that help activate immune responses.

Lymphatic tissues:

a. Lymphoid follicles: Clusters of lymphocytes in various parts of the body, such as the spleen and lymph nodes.

b. Mucosa-associated lymphoid tissue (MALT): lymphoid tissue found on mucous membranes such as the respiratory, gastrointestinal, and genitourinary tracts.

These organs and tissues work together to help protect the body from infection, disease, and other foreign substances.

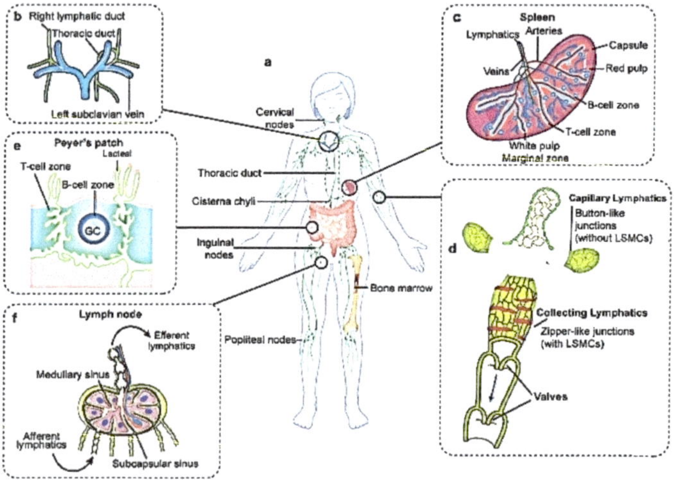

Fig. 49. Lymphatic vessels.

2.2. Lymphatic vessels:

Lymphatic vessels are a key part of the lymphatic system, responsible for transporting lymph throughout the body.

I. Types of lymphatic vessels:

i. Lymphatic capillaries: The smallest lymphatic vessels that absorb interstitial fluid (fluid between cells) from tissues.

ii. Medium-sized lymphatic collection vessels collect lymph from capillaries and transport it to larger vessels.

iii. Lymphatic trunks: These are large vessels that receive lymphatic fluid from collecting vessels and transport it to lymph nodes or other lymphatic organs.

iv. Lymphatic ducts: These are the largest lymphatic vessels that empty lymph into the bloodstream.

II. Importance of lymphatic vessels:

a. One-way valves: prevent lymph backflow and ensure that it moves in one direction to the lymph nodes or other lymph organs.

b. Thin walls: Allow lymphatic vessels the flexibility needed to accommodate varying amounts of fluid.

c. Smooth muscle, found in larger lymphatic vessels, helps propel lymph through contraction.

III. Functions of lymphatic vessels:

i. Fluid transport: Lymphatic vessels transport lymph from the tissues back into the circulation.

ii. Protein transport: Lymphatic vessels help return proteins lost from blood vessels back into circulation.

IV. Main lymphatic vessels:

a. Thoracic duct: The largest lymphatic vessel that drains most of the body (except the right side of the head, neck, chest, and right arm) into the bloodstream. The right lymphatic duct drains the right side of the head, neck, chest, and right arm.

b. Cisterna chyli: An enlarged lymphatic vessel located in front of the L1-L2 vertebrae that receives lymphatic fluid from the lower extremities, these vessels play a vital role in maintaining fluid balance, immune function, and overall health.

2.3. Mechanisms of lymph circulation:

I. Several mechanisms help facilitate lymph circulation:

i. Skeletal muscle contractions Skeletal muscle contractions compress and decompress lymphatic vessels, forcing fluid forward.

ii. Breathing Movements: While breathing, diaphragmatic contractions also compress and decompress the thoracic duct to aid fluid movement.

The lymphatic system plays a crucial role in lymph circulation:

a. Lymphatic circulation: The lymph's through the body consists of several steps:

i. Formation of interstitial fluid: Fluid leaks from blood capillaries into the interstitial spaces between cells.

ii. Lymphatic capillary absorption: The lymphatic capillaries absorb the interstitial fluid.

iii. Transport by lymphatic vessels: Lymphatic fluid is transported by collecting vessels to larger trunks.

iv. Lymph node filtration: One or more sets of lymph nodes filter lymph fluid for pathogens and other foreign substances.
v. Lymphatic Drainage: The thoracic duct, also known as the right lymphatic duct, empties the filtered lymphatic fluid into the bloodstream.

II. Factors affecting lymph circulation:
Several factors can affect lymph circulation:
i. Exercise: Regular exercise can help improve muscle contractions and lymph circulation.
ii. Breathing techniques: Deep breathing exercises can help compress and decompress the chest canal.
iii. Maintaining proper posture can reduce thoracic duct compression and improve fluid flow.
iv. The complex network of the lymphatic system plays a vital role in maintaining our overall health.

2.4. Functions of lymphatic system:
The lymphatic system plays a vital role in maintaining overall health by performing several critical functions:
a. Maintaining fluid balance: Returns interstitial fluid to the bloodstream to ensure proper blood volume and pressure.
b. Protein conservation helps return proteins lost from blood vessels back into circulation.
c. Supporting immune function provides a network for immune cells (lymphocytes) to move around the body and respond to infections.
d. Waste Removal: Removes waste products from tissues, such as excess proteins, bacteria, viruses, and dead cells.
e. Infection Prevention: Activates immune responses to prevent infections from spreading throughout the body.
f. Cancer cell removal: Helps remove cancer cells from tissues before they can spread to other parts of the body.
g. Absorption of nutrients: It plays a role in the absorption of fats and fat-soluble vitamins from the digestive tract into the bloodstream.

Related questions from unit 3

1. Elaborate in detail about blood coagulation.
2. Describe in brief about anaemia.
3. Describe in brief about lymphatic tissue.
4. Explain in brief about blood transfusion.
5. Explain the Rh factor with its significance.
6. Explain in brief about the composition of blood with its functions.
7. Explain in detail about blood circulation.
8. Explain the intrinsic pathway of blood coagulation.
9. Explain the types of blood vessels.
10. Write in detail blood grouping system and Rh factors?
11. Describe the blood clotting pathway.
12. Explain in detail the reticular endothelial cell.
13. Elaborate the term blood pressure in detail.
14. Describe the components of lymphatic circulation in detail.
15. Explain the disorders of lymphatic gland and lymph nodes.

Unit – 4.

Topic	Page no.
Chapter 1: Peripheral nervous system	110 – 111
1.1. Classification of peripheral nervous system	111 – 114
1.2. The structure and functions of the sympathetic and parasympathetic nervous system	114 – 116
1.3. Origin and functions of spinal and cranial nerves	116 – 118

Topic	Page no.
Chapter 2: Special senses	119 – 120
2.1. Structure and functions of eye	120 – 121
2.2. Disorder of eye	121 – 122
2.3. Structure and functions of ear	122 – 124
2.4. Disorder of ear	124 – 126
2.5. Structure and functions of nose	126 – 127
2.6. Disorder of nose	127 – 128
2.7. Structure and functions of tongue	128 – 129
2.8. Disorder of tongue	129 – 131

Related questions from unit 4	132

Unit – 4.

Chapter 1.
Peripheral Nervous System.

The peripheral nervous system (PNS) is an essential component of our nervous system that links our brain and spinal cord to the remaining parts of our body.

The peripheral nervous system (PNS) comprises a network of nerves that establish connections between our central nervous system (CNS), encompassing the brain and spinal cord, to our limbs, organs, and senses. It is responsible for facilitating the transmission of information between our central nervous system (CNS) and our peripheral organs.

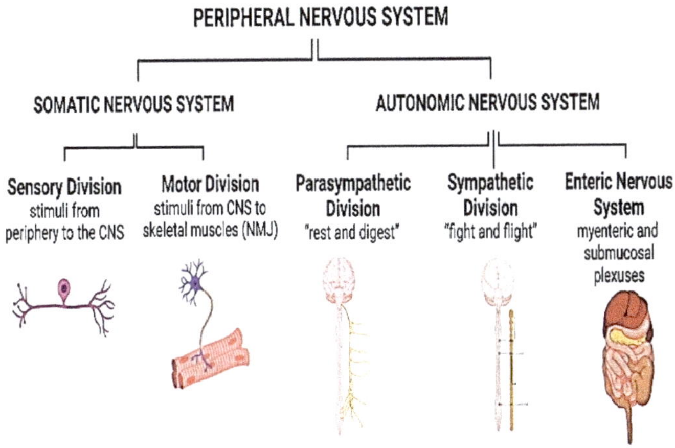

Fig. 50. Peripheral nervous system types.

The peripheral nervous system performs the following functions:

a. Sensory input: process sensory stimuli from the environment, including tactile sensations, temperature, nociception, and vibrations.

b. Motor output refers to the transmission of motor impulses from our central nervous system (CNS) to our muscles or glands, regulation refers to the control and coordination of numerous body activities, such as heart rate, digestion, and circulation.

The peripheral nervous system's subdivisions include:

There are two primary subdivisions that make up the peripheral nervous system (PNS).
i. The somatic nervous system is responsible for regulating voluntary movements of skeletal muscles.
ii. The Autonomic Nervous System (ANS) controls the involuntary activities of smooth muscle, cardiac muscle, and glands.

Subdivisions of the Autonomic Nervous System: we further divided the ANS into two subdivisions:
a. The Sympathetic Nervous System (SNS) activates our body's stress reaction, known as the fight-or-flight response.
b. The Parasympathetic Nervous System (PNS) facilitates relaxation, recuperation, and conservation of energy.

Peripheral nerve anatomy: Peripheral nerves consist of numerous layers.
i. Axon: A slender and elongated projection of a neuron that transmits signals away from the cell body towards the synapse.
ii. The myelin sheath is a fatty layer that surrounds the axon and helps to enhance the passage of signals.
iii. The neurilemma is a thin layer of connective tissue that surrounds and maintains the myelin sheath of a nerve fiber.
iv. The endoneurium is a thin layer of connective tissue that surrounds a nerve fiber and keeps it in place.

Peripheral Nervous System diseases and disorders: Numerous diseases and disorders can impact the peripheral nervous system (PNS), including neuropathy, a medical condition.
a. Multiple sclerosis is a medical condition characterized by damage to the protective covering of nerve fibers in the central nervous system.
b. Guillain-Barré syndrome is a medical condition.
c. Injury to nerves that are not part of the brain or spinal cord

1.1. Peripheral nervous system classification:
Depending on its function, the peripheral nervous system (PNS) falls into two primary classifications:
a. The Somatic Nervous System (SNS) is the part of the peripheral nervous system that controls voluntary movements and sensory perception; the somatic nervous system regulates voluntary movements of skeletal muscles through the inclusion of motor neurons that convey impulses to the skeletal muscles, the sensory nerves are responsible for transmitting messages. Sensory receptors Integumentary system, articulations, and muscular system

b. The Autonomic Nervous System (ANS) is a part of the peripheral nervous system that controls involuntary bodily functions, the autonomic nervous system controls voluntary bodily activities. Smooth muscle, heart muscle, and glands. The inclusion of both sympathetic and parasympathetic divisions.

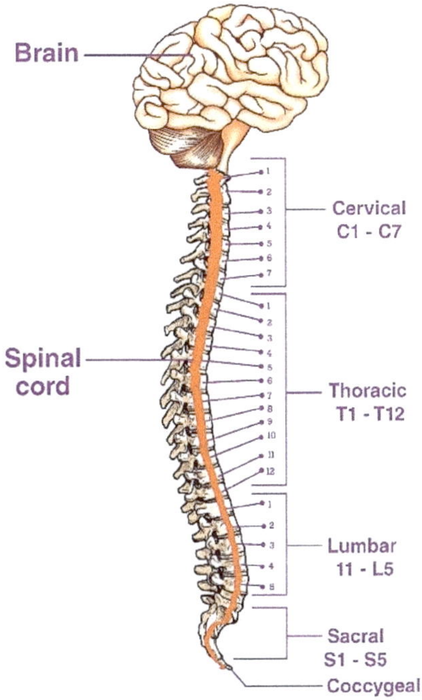

Fig. 51. The Brain and spinal cord.

I. Structural based classification:

Depending on its structure, we can also divide the peripheral nervous system (PNS) into two primary classifications: Cranial nerve and Spinal nerve.

A. Cranial Nerves: The brainstem is the point of origin that regulates a range of functions in the head and neck, including sensory and motor processes, there are 12 pairs of cranial nerves.

a. Olfactory nerve: A sensory nerve that carries olfactory stimuli from the nasal cavity to the brain which stimulate the sense of smell (Cranial nerve-I).

b. Optic nerve: The second pair of cranial nerves facilitates the transmission of impulses from the retina in the posterior eye to the brain (Cranial nerve-II).
c. Oculomotor nerve: It is a bilateral nerve responsible for regulating eye movement, pupil constriction, and eyelid retraction (Cranial nerve-III).
d. Trochlear nerve: It enables movement in your eye's superior oblique muscle (Cranial nerve-IV).
e. Trigeminal nerve: It has three main branches: ophthalmic, maxillary, and mandibular (Cranial nerve-V).
f. Abducens nerve: Controls a muscle that moves the eyeball (Cranial nerve-VI).
g. Facial nerve: Supplies the muscles of facial expression (Cranial nerve-VII).
h. Vestibulocochlear nerve: It is responsible for hearing and balance (Cranial nerve-VIII).
i. Glossopharyngeal nerve: It has both sensory and motor functions, including providing a sense of taste for the back of the tongue, and stimulating a muscle in the back of the throat (Cranial nerve-IX).
j. Vagus nerve: Enervates the heart, larynx, and gut (Cranial nerve-X).
k. Accessory nerve: Energizes the sternocleidomastoid and trapezius muscles (Cranial nerve-XI).
l. Hypoglossal: Enervates the muscles of the tongue (Cranial nerve-XII).

B. Spinal Nerves: The spinal cord originates from the brainstem, it regulates a multitude of bodily systems, including sensory and motor functions. There are 31 pairs of spinal nerves:

II. Distribution based classification:
Depending on its distribution, we can also divide the peripheral nervous system (PNS) into two primary classifications: The central nervous system (CNS) consists of the brain and spinal cord, whereas the peripheral nervous system (PNS) includes all the nerves outside of the CNS, the nervous system consists of nerves that begin from the brainstem and spinal cord and spread throughout the central section of the body. Nerves make up the peripheral nervous system, the nervous system includes nerves that originate in the peripheral areas of the body and distribute to other peripheral parts of the body.

III. Classification based on innervation: It refers to categorizing anything according to the nerves that supply it, based on its innervation, we can also categorize the peripheral nervous system (PNS) into two primary groups.

i. Somatic innervation refers to the nerve supply that controls voluntary movements and sensations in the body. It transmits information to the nerves responsible for innervating skeletal muscles, skin, and joints.
ii. Visceral Innervation: The text includes information about the nerves that provide innervation to smooth muscle, cardiac muscle, and glands.

1.2. The structure and functions of the sympathetic and parasympathetic nervous system:

The anatomical organization and physiological roles of the sympathetic and parasympathetic divisions of the autonomic nervous system are the focus of discussion. These two systems are components of the autonomous nervous system, which regulates involuntary physiological activities. there are two primary divisions that make up the Autonomic Nervous System (ANS):

a) The Sympathetic Nervous System (SNS)
b) The Parasympathetic Nervous System (PNS)

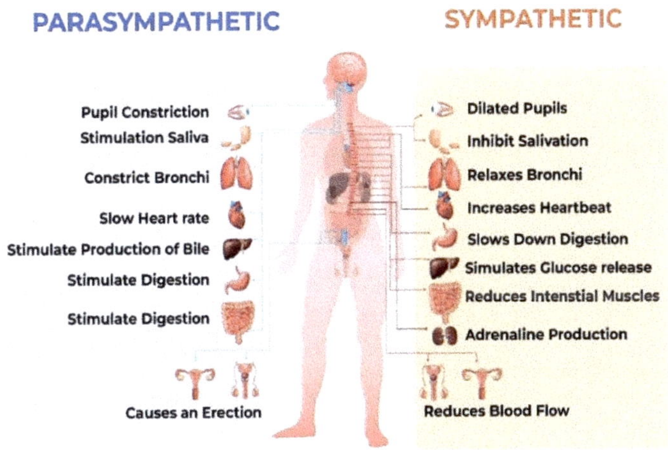

Fig. 52. Sympathetic and parasympathetic activity.

A. The Sympathetic Nervous System (SNS) forms:

i. The spinal cord arises from the thoracic and lumbar segments.
ii. The system employs short preganglionic fibers and elongated postganglionic fibers.
iii. The spinal cord and ganglia are in close proximity.
iv. The main neurotransmitter used by most neurons is norepinephrine, with the exception of sweat glands, which utilize acetylcholine.

Functions:
a. Frequently referred to as the "fight or flight" system
b. It facilitates physiological adaptations to cope with stressful or emergency situations.
c. The medication elevates heart rate and raises blood pressure.
d. Causes pupil dilation
e. Elevates respiratory rate
f. Redirects blood circulation towards skeletal muscles and essential organs
g. Induces perspiration
h. Reduces gastrointestinal and renal functions

B. The Parasympathetic Nervous System (PNS) forms:
The brainstem, specifically the cranial nerves III, VII, IX, and X, and the sacral portion of the spinal cord cause this phenomenon, use long preganglionic fibers and abbreviated or short postganglionic fibers.
The target organs are in close proximity to or contain ganglia.
Acetylcholine is the main or primary neurotransmitter.

Functions:
a. Commonly referred to as the "rest and digest" or "feed and breed" method.
b. It facilitates relaxation and fosters the preservation of energy.
c. Reduces heart rate and lowers blood pressure
d. Causes pupil constriction
e. Improves gastrointestinal and urinary system function.
f. Enhances sexual stimulation
g. It stimulates salivary production.
h. Reduces the frequency of respiration.

Notable distinctions or differences:
a. Origin: The somatic nervous system originates from the thoracolumbar area, whereas the peripheral nervous system originates from the craniosacral region.
b. Fiber length: The sympathetic nervous system (SNS) is characterized by short preganglionic fibers and lengthy postganglionic fibers, whereas the parasympathetic nervous system (PNS) has the opposite pattern.
c. Location: In the sympathetic nervous system (SNS), the ganglion is located near the spinal cord, and in the parasympathetic nervous system (PNS), it is located near or inside the target organs.
d. Neurotransmitters: The sympathetic nervous system (SNS) predominantly utilizes norepinephrine, whereas the parasympathetic nervous system (PNS) employs acetylcholine.

e. Effects: The sympathetic nervous system (SNS) normally produces excitatory responses, whereas the parasympathetic nervous system (PNS) generally produces inhibitory responses, but there are occasional exceptions.

f. Collaboration: The sympathetic nervous system (SNS) and parasympathetic nervous system (PNS) sometimes operate in opposition to sustain equilibrium (Homeostasis) inside the body. for example:

i. The sympathetic nervous system (SNS) elevates heart rate, whereas the parasympathetic nervous system (PNS) reduces it.

ii. The sympathetic nervous system (SNS) causes the pupils to expand, while the parasympathetic nervous system (PNS) causes them to contract.

iii. The sympathetic nervous system (SNS) hinders the process of digestion, whereas the parasympathetic nervous system (PNS) promotes it.

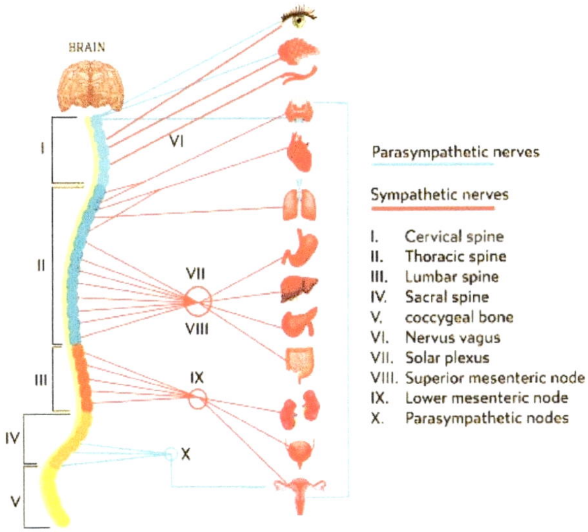

Fig. 53. Origin and function of spinal and cranial nerves.

1.3. The origin and function of the spinal and cranial nerves:

The origins and function of spinal and cranial nerves are the focus of discussion, it is divided into two components: spinal nerves and cranial nerves.

a. Spinal nerves:

i. Source: The spinal cord is where spinal nerves originate, in humans, there are a total of 31 pairs of spinal nerves that exit the spinal cord through the intervertebral foramina, which are holes located between the vertebrae.

ii. Functionalities: Spinal nerves provide both sensory and motor capabilities. We classify these nerves as mixed because they comprise both sensory (afferent) and motor (efferent) nerve fibers.

iii. Sensory functions: Sensory neurons transmit sensory information from different regions of the body to the central nervous system (CNS), these sensations encompass tactile, compressive, thermal, and nociceptive stimuli.

iv. Motor function: Motor neurons transmit motor signals from the central nervous system (CNS) to muscles, regulating voluntary movements.

v. Autonomic function: Certain fibers are involved in the autonomic nerve system, regulating involuntary physiological processes such as heart rate, digestion, and blood pressure.

Spinal Nerves: Depending on the specific region of the spine from which they originate, the spinal nerves fall into one of five distinct categories:

i. The cervical region of the spine consists of 8 pairs of vertebrae.

ii. The thoracic vertebrae consist of 12 pairs of vertebrae.

iii. The lumbar region of the spine consists of 5 pairs of vertebrae.

iv. Sacral region it consists of 5 pairs of vertebrae.

v. Coccygeal (1 pair) refers to the presence of one pair of coccygeal bones.

b. Cranial nerves:

i. Source: The cranial nerves have their genesis in the brain and brainstem. In humans, there are a total of 12 pairs of cranial nerves that emerge straight from the skull through different holes called foramina.

ii. Functions: Cranial nerves exhibit a wide range of functions, and in contrast to spinal nerves, not all cranial nerves possess both sensory and motor components. Some neurons are solely responsible for sensory functions, some for motor functions, and others have a combination of both, the followings are the main function:

i. Olfactory refers to the sense of smell.

ii. The optic nerve is a sensory nerve responsible for vision.

iii. The oculomotor nerve regulates eye movement and pupil constriction.
iv. The trochlear nerve, which regulates eye movement, activates the superior oblique muscle.
v. The trigeminal nerve is a mixed nerve that is responsible for both facial sensibility and chewing muscle control.
vi. The lateral rectus muscle activates the abducens nerve, which controls the movement of the eye.
vii. Facial: This cranial nerve is responsible for a combination of functions, including facial expressions, taste perception, and control of certain glands.
viii. The vestibulocochlear nerve is responsible for sensory functions related to hearing and balance.
xi. The glossopharyngeal nerve is a mixed nerve that carries signals related to taste, throat feeling, and certain glands.
x. The vagus nerve has mixed innervation, supplying various organs.
xi. Accessory: Muscles of the neck.
xii. The hypoglossal nerve is responsible for tongue motion-related motor functions.

Distinctive disparities or differences exist between spinal and cranial nerves:

a. Spinal nerves originate in the spinal cord, whereas cranial nerves originate in the brain and brainstem.
b. There are a total of 31 pairs of spinal nerves and 12 pairs of cranial nerves.
c. Nomenclature: The exact segment of the spinal cord from which a spinal nerve originates or placed determines its designation, while cranial nerves receive roman numerals as according to their positions and have unique names.
d. Regarding function specificity, it is important to note that whereas all spinal nerves have both sensory and motor functions, cranial nerves might have either sensory, motor, or a combination of both.

Unit – 4.

Chapter 2.
Special Senses.

Special senses: These are a group of sensory systems that provide us with specific types of information about our environment. These senses are distinct from the general senses (like touch) and include: vision (sight), audition (hearing), gustation (taste), olfaction (smell), equilibrium, or homeostasis (balance and touch).

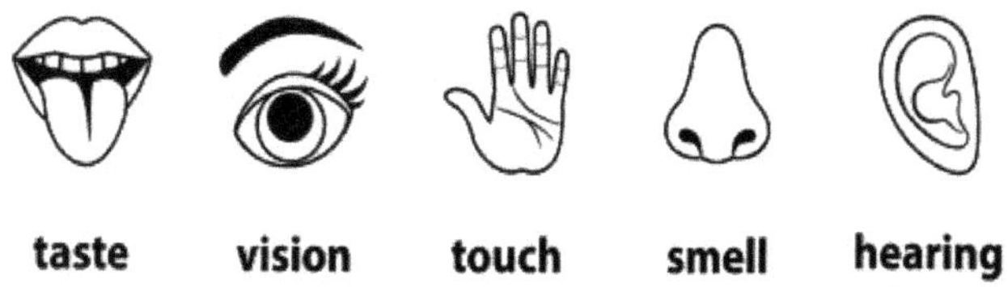

Fig 54. Special senses.

The special senses are:
i. Vision (sight):
Organ location: Eyes.
Function: Detects light and colour, allowing us to perceive the visual world.
Key structures: retina, lens, cornea, optic nerve.

ii. Audition (Hearing):
Organ location: Ears.
Function: Detects sound waves, enabling us to perceive sounds.
Key structures: cochlea, auditory ossicles, eardrum.

iii. Gustation (Taste):

Organ location: Tongue.
Function: Detects chemical compounds in food, allowing us to perceive taste.
Key structures: taste buds, papillae.

iv. Olfaction (Smell):
Organ location: Nose.
Function: Detects airborne chemicals, allowing us to perceive odours.
Key structures: olfactory epithelium, olfactory bulb.

v. Equilibrium or homeostasis (balance):
Organ location: Inner ear.
Function: Detects head position and movement, ensuring balance.
Key structures: semi-circular canals, vestibule.

Each of these special senses works through specialized receptor cells that convert specific stimuli into electrical signals, the brain processes and interprets these signals, enabling us to perceive and interact with our environment.

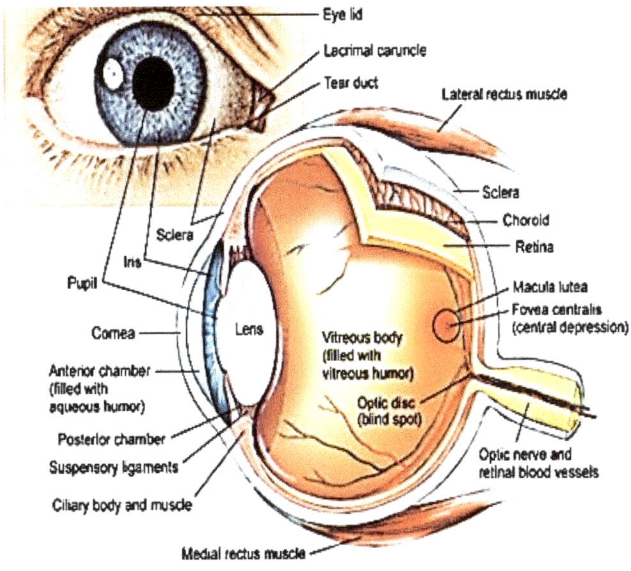

Fig. 55. Structure of human eye.

A. Eye:

2.1. Structure and functions of the eye: The human eye is a complex and fascinating organ that allows us to perceive the visual world around us.

Structure of the eye:

i. Cornea: The transparent, dome-shaped surface located in front of the eye.
ii. Iris: The coloured part of the eye that controls the amount of light entering.
iii. Pupil: The dark center of the iris that allows light to enter the eye.
iv. Lens: A clear, flexible structure behind the iris that directs light onto the retina.
v. Retina: The light-sensitive layer at the back of the eye containing photoreceptor cells.
vi. Optic Nerve: The nerve that carries visual information from the retina to the brain.
vii. Sclera: The white, protective outer layer of the eyeball.
viii. Choroid: A layer of blood vessels between the sclera and retina that provides nutrients.
ix. Vitreous humours: A clear, gel-like substance that fills the space between the lens and retina.
x. Aqueous humours: a clear fluid in the front part of the eye that maintains eye pressure.

Functions of the eye:

i. Light reception: The cornea and lens focus light onto the retina.
ii. Light regulation: To control the amount of light entering the eye, the iris adjusts the size of the pupil.
iii. Image formation: The lens focuses light to produce a clear image on the retina.
iv. Photoreception: Rod and cone cells in the retina convert light into electrical signals.
v. Signal transmission: The optic nerve sends visual information to the brain for processing.
vi. Colour perception: Cone cells allow us to see different colours.
vii. Dark Adaptation: Rod cells help us see in low-light conditions.
viii. Depth perception: Both eyes work together to provide stereoscopic vision.
ix. Eye Protection: Eyelids, eyelashes, and tear production protect the eye from damage and keep it moist.
x. Eye Movement: The muscles attached to the eye allow for precise movements and object tracking.

2.2. Disorders of the eye: The eye is a complex organ, and there are numerous disorders that can affect its function and health. Let's go through some of the most common eye disorders:

a. Refractive errors: myopia (near-sightedness), hyperopia (farsightedness), astigmatism Age-related difficulty focusing on close objects is known as presbyopia.

b. cataracts: A clouding of the eye's natural lens, leading to blurred vision.

c. Glaucoma: A group of eye conditions that damage the optic nerve, often due to increased intraocular pressure.

d. Age-related Macular Degeneration (AMD): A condition affecting the central part of the retina (macula), causing loss of central vision.

e. Diabetic retinopathy: diabetes-related damage to the blood vessels in the retina.

f. Dry eye syndrome: Insufficient tear production or rapid tear evaporation, leading to eye discomfort and irritation.

g. Conjunctivitis: inflammation of the conjunctiva, often caused by infection or allergies.

h. Retinal Detachment: separation of the retina from the back of the eye, which can lead to vision loss if not treated promptly.

i. Amblyopia (lazy eye): reduced vision in one eye due to abnormal visual development in childhood.

j. Strabismus causes eyes to look in different directions. uveitis refers to an inflammation of the uvea, which is the middle layer of the eye.

l. Keratoconus: A progressive thinning and bulging of the cornea.

m. Retinitis Pigmentosa: A group of inherited disorders that cause progressive vision loss.

n. Ocular migraines: temporary visual disturbances, sometimes accompanied by headaches.

o. Colour blindness: The inability to distinguish between specific colours, usually inherited.

These disorders can vary in severity and impact on vision. While ongoing Proper medical care and management may be necessary to prevent further vision loss in others, regular eye exams are crucial for early detection and treatment of eye disorders.

b. Ear:

2.3. Structure and functions of the ear:

The anatomy and physiological processes of the ear: They are the intricate and captivating organ that has a vital function in human auditory perception and equilibrium maintenance.

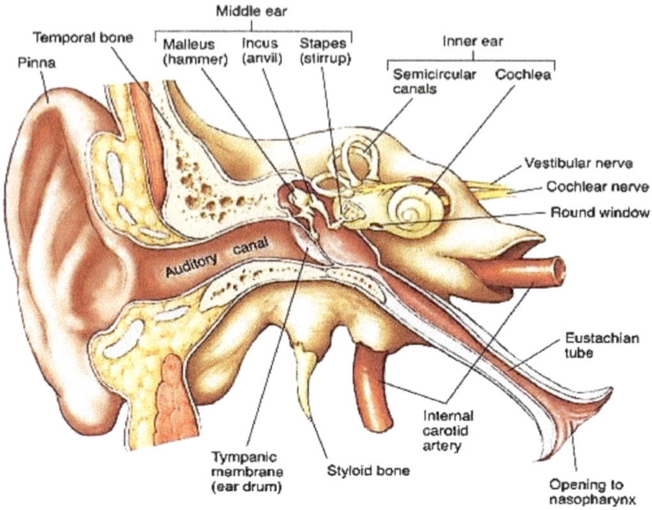

Fig. 56. Structure of human ear.

Structure of the ear: The ear is anatomically comprised of three primary components:

a. Auricle:

i. Pinna (auricle): The externally visible portion of the ear responsible for gathering sound waves.

ii. The ear canal, also known as the external auditory meatus, is a tube that connects to the eardrum.

iii. Tympanic membrane (eardrum): A delicate membrane that oscillates in reaction to sound waves.

b. The middle ear:

i. Ossicles: The auditory system consists of three minuscule bones known as the malleus (hammer), incus (anvil), and stapes (stirrup).

ii. The Eustachian tube serves to establish equilibrium in air pressure by connecting the middle ear to the posterior part of the throat.

c. Cochlea:

i. Cochlea: A spiral-shaped, liquid-filled organ that is responsible for the sense of hearing, the semi-circular canals consist of three fluid-filled loops that aid in maintaining equilibrium.
iii. Vestibule: The vestibule houses the utricle and saccule, which are both important in maintaining equilibrium.

Function of the ear:
The primary function of the ear is to facilitate the sense of hearing.
i. The external ear gathers sound waves and directs them into the ear canal towards the eardrum.
ii. The tympanic membrane oscillates in reaction to acoustic waves.
iii. The ossicles within the middle ear enhance and convey these vibrations to the inner ear.
iv. Hair cells in the cochlea transform vibrations into electrical messages. these impulses are sent to the brain through the auditory nerve, where they are perceived as sound.

Equilibrium and Spatial Orientation:
i. The semi-circular canals perceive rotational motions of the head.
ii. the utricle and saccule, located in the vestibule, perceive linear acceleration and determine the location of the head in relation to gravity.
iii. The brain receives this information in order to preserve equilibrium and spatial perception.

Equalization of pressure:
The Eustachian tube facilitates the equalization of air pressure between the middle ear and the external environment, a crucial process for maintaining healthy eardrum function.
a. Protection: The anatomical structure of the outer ear and the presence of earwax (cerumen) serve to safeguard the ear against foreign objects, dust, and bacteria.
b. Sound localization: The brain utilizes minute disparities in the timing and amplitude of sounds reaching each ear to ascertain the direction of sound origins.
Gaining knowledge about the anatomy and operations of the ear allows us to recognize the intricacy of our auditory system and the significance of safeguarding our hearing well-being.

2.4. Disorder of ear: The ear is an intricate organ that is important for both hearing and balance, and it can be impacted by a range of illnesses.
i. Otitis Media (Middle Ear illness): This is a prevalent illness, particularly in youngsters, common symptoms encompass otalgia,

pyrexia, and transient auditory impairment. The condition might arise due to viral or bacterial pathogens.

ii. Tinnitus: A medical disorder characterized by the perception of ringing, buzzing, or other auditory sensations in the ear, the condition might arise due to the exposure to high decibel sounds, age-related auditory decline, or several other contributing factors.

iii. Meniere's Disease: A condition affecting the inner ear that can result in dizziness, loss of hearing, and ringing in the ears. The condition is believed to be caused by an accumulation of fluid in the inner ear.

iv. Acoustic Neuroma: A benign tumour that forms on the nerve that links the ear to the brain, it can result in auditory impairment, equilibrium issues, and the perception of ringing in the ears.

v. Presbycusis is a term used to describe the progressive loss of hearing that happens as a person becomes older, primarily it first impacts high-frequency noises.

vi. Cerumen Impaction: The accumulation of an excessive amount of cerumen (ear wax) can lead to auditory difficulties and pain.

vii. Labyrinthitis: Inflammation of the inner ear resulting in vertigo and hearing impairment.

Frequently triggered by viral illnesses.

a. Otosclerosis is a genetic disorder characterized by aberrant bone development in the middle ear, leading to hearing loss.

b. Perichondritis: A condition characterized by the infection of the cartilage in the outer ear, typically resulting from damage or piercing.

c. Cholesteatoma: A pathological proliferation of skin cells in the middle ear that has the potential to cause harm to nearby anatomical structures.

d. Vestibular Neuritis: Inflammation of the vestibular nerve, resulting in severe vertigo.

e. Ear barotrauma refers to the damage caused to the ear as a result of alterations in air or water pressure, which is frequently experienced during air travel or diving.

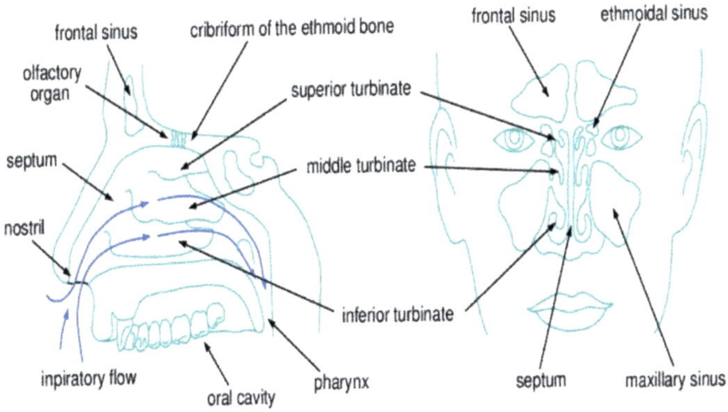

Fig. 57. Structure of human nose.

C. Nose: The nose consists of various structures and carries out various functions. The nose is an essential component of our respiratory system and fulfils several crucial functions.

2.5. Structure and functions of the nose:

Structure:

a. Nasal External: The integumentary system envelops the structure, which consists of osseous and cartilaginous tissues and features a pair of nares (nostrils) divided by the nasal septum.

i. Internal Nose: The nasal septum divides the nasal cavity into separate left and right chambers.

ii. Nasal conchae (turbinate's): osseous protrusions that augment the extent of the surface area.

iii. The paranasal sinuses are air-filled cavities in the skull that connect to the nasal cavity.

iv. The superior portion of the nasal cavity houses the olfactory area; the respiratory area is located in the bottom section of the nose cavity.

Functions:

i. Respiration serves as the primary pathway for the breathing process.

ii. This process's function is to filter, heat, and add moisture to the air that enters the system. Additionally, it is responsible for the sense of smell.

iii. The olfactory receptors are located in the superior region of the nasal cavity, this organ perceives, aids in the perception of smells, and enhances the sensation of taste.

iv. Filtration is the process of passing solid particles from a liquid or gas by passing it through a porous material or medium, Nasal hairs, also

known as vibrissae, and mucus serve to ensnare dust, allergies, and other particles.
iv. Air conditioning helps to prevent hazardous chemicals from entering the lungs, the function is to raise the temperature and moisture level of the breathed air to match the body's temperature, achieving almost 100% humidity, it assists in protecting the delicate tissues of the lungs.
v. Vocal resonance: It serves as a resonant cavity, enhancing the quality of your vocalization.
vi. Drainage: It facilitates the flow of tears via the nasolacrimal duct, removes surplus mucus from the paranasal sinuses.
vii. Immune system protection: The substance contains immune cells that aid in the defences against harmful microorganisms.
viii. Production of Nitric Oxide: It generates nitric oxide, which has antibacterial characteristics and aids in the regulation of pulmonary blood circulation. The intricate anatomy of the nose enables it to efficiently carry out a wide range of duties, making it a vital component of our respiratory and sensory systems. The filtration, warming, and humidification of air before it enters our lungs is essential for preserving respiratory well-being.

2.6. Disorder of nose: Those are conditions that affect the nose, a range of illnesses can influence the nose, a vital component of our respiratory system. Now, let's check into a few prevalent nasal disorders:
i. Rhinitis: Allergies or factors unrelated to allergies can cause rhinitis, which is the inflammation of the nasal passages, common symptoms encompass nasal discharge, frequent sneezing, and nasal congestion.
ii. Sinusitis: The medical term for the inflammation or swelling of the tissue lining the sinuses is sinusitis. The condition can manifest as either acute or chronic and presents symptoms such as face discomfort, nasal discharge, and diminished olfactory perception.
iii. Deviated septum: It refers to the displacement of the thin wall (septum) between the nasal passages, resulting in one nasal tube being smaller than the other.
iv. Nasal polyps: They are benign growths that can form in the nasal passages or sinuses. They are soft, painless, and noncancerous.
v. Nosebleeds (Epistaxis): It is often known as nosebleeds, refers to the occurrence of bleeding from the nose. Several factors, including dry air, physical injury, or specific drugs, can cause this.
vi. Nasal fractures are the result of trauma or injury, causing the nose's bones to break.
vii. Rhinophyma: It is a medical disorder characterized by the appearance of a prominent, red, and swollen nose. People with severe rosacea commonly exhibit it.

viii. Nasal tumours are benign or cancerous growths that are located in the nasal cavity or paranasal sinuses.

ix. Anosmia: It refers to the absence or loss of the sense of smell. Several sources, such as viral infections, head injuries, or the natural process of aging, can cause this condition to occur either temporarily or permanently.

x. Nasal valve collapse refers to a structural issue that may cause difficulties in nasal breathing.

xi. Atrophic rhinitis: It is a chronic illness characterized by the gradual degeneration of the nasal mucosa, resulting in malodorous nasal discharge and crust formation.

xii. Choanal atresia: It is a congenital disorder characterized by an obstruction of the posterior nasal passage, typically caused by aberrant bone or soft tissue.

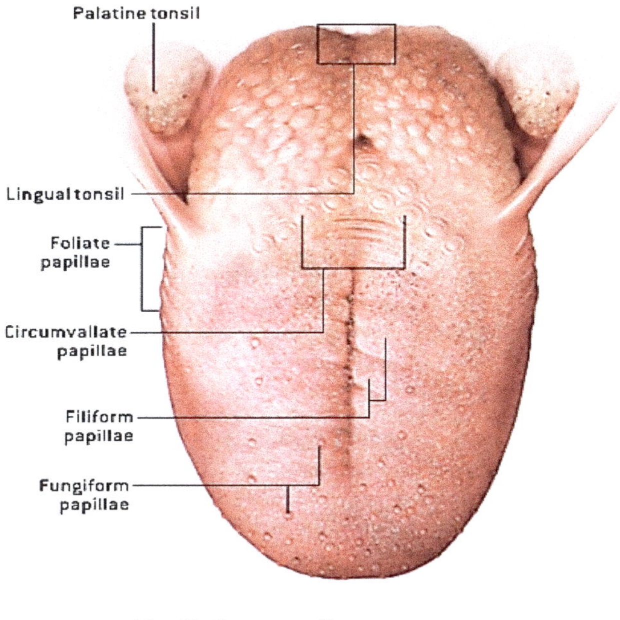

Fig. 58. Structure of human tongue.

D. Tongue: The tongue (to taste) is an intriguing and necessary organ in our body, fulfilling vital functions in numerous facets of our everyday existence. Now, let's check the composition and roles of this entity. The majority of the tongue is made up of skeletal muscles, both intrinsic (found inside the tongue) and extrinsic (found connected to other tissues).

2.7. Structure and functions of the tongue:

Structure: A mucous membrane coats the tongue, papillae are minute elevated formations on the tongue's surface that house taste receptors. There exist four distinct types:

a. Filiform papillae are the most abundant type of papillae found on the tongue, and they are responsible for its coarse texture.

b. Fungiform papillae: Distributed throughout the thread-like papillae are taste buds.

c. Circumvallate papillae: The tongue's posterior region displays larger papillae arranged in a V-shaped pattern.

d. Foliate papillae: Located on the lateral aspects of the tongue.

Taste buds: They are sensory cell agglomerations that are responsible for flavour perception.

Those nerves extensively supply the tongue, serving both to transmit sensory information and to govern its movements. The tongue relies on a well-developed network of blood vessels to maintain its appropriate functioning and overall health.

Function:

The tongue has the following functions:

i. Taste: The main role of taste buds on the tongue is to perceive five fundamental tastes: sweet, sour, salty, bitter, and umami.

ii. Speech: It relies heavily on the tongue, since it plays a vital role in producing sounds and shaping words, making it an indispensable component of communication.

iii. Mastication: This also known as chewing, facilitates the manipulation of food within the oral cavity and shapes it into a cohesive mass called a bolus, which may then be swallowed.

iv. Swallowing: To trigger the swallowing response, the tongue propels food toward the posterior part of the throat.

v. Cleaning: It helps remove food debris from the mouth and teeth, promoting oral hygiene.

vi. Temperature and texture sensing: The tongue has the ability to perceive and distinguish the temperature and texture of food and beverages.

vii. Saliva distribution: It allows saliva to disperse throughout the oral cavity, which helps with digestion and oral hygiene maintenance.
viii. Communication: The tongue can make facial expressions or gestures in some cultural contexts.
ix. Immune Function: The tongue contains lymphoid tissue that contributes to the immunological function of the oral cavity.

2.8. Disorder of tongue: Tongue disorders can present in several ways, such as alterations in colour, texture, size, and mobility. A variety of factors, including infections, dietary deficiencies, and systemic illnesses, can cause these problems.

Common tongue disorders:
1. Glossitis: The tongue is inflamed, causing it to expand, change colour and become painful. It may arise from infections, allergic responses, or nutritional insufficiencies, namely a deficiency in vitamins B12, iron, or folate. Treatment often entails treating the root cause, such as enhancing nutritional intake or employing topical treatments to alleviate symptoms.

2. Melanoglossia: This disorder, known as lingua villosa nigra, arises when necrotic cells and bacteria build on the surface of the tongue, resulting in a black and hairy look. People frequently attribute it to poor dental hygiene, tobacco use, or certain drugs. Enhancing oral hygiene practices often resolves the problem.

3. Fissured or cracked tongue: A fissured tongue is characterized by the presence of grooves or fissures on its surface, and it is often benign. It might be associated with hereditary factors or situations, such as geographic tongue. Although there is no need for a special treatment, it is crucial to maintain proper oral hygiene in order to avoid discomfort and infection.

4. Geographic Tongue (Condition of the tongue's Surface): This innocent illness manifests as sleek, crimson spots on the tongue around pale perimeters, mimicking a cartographic representation. It may cause discomfort or sensitivity, but it typically does not require treatment unless the symptoms are severe.

5. Burning mouth syndrome: It is a medical condition characterized by a sensation of burning pain in the mouth, this illness is characterized by a continuous sensation of burning in the tongue and mouth. It might be associated with hormonal shifts, dietary deficits, or psychological

problems. The treatment may entail addressing the root causes and using drugs to alleviate symptoms.

6. Macroglossia (Enlarged tongue): Macroglossia is the medical term for an abnormally big tongue, which can be present from birth (congenital) or develop later in life (acquired). Disorders such as Down syndrome, acromegaly, and certain cancers can link to it. Treatment frequently focuses on effectively controlling the root cause, and in more severe cases, surgical interventions may be required.

7. Candidiasis of the oral cavity (Oral thrush): Candida causes candidiasis, a fungal illness that can cause white spots on the tongue and throughout the oral cavity. It is particularly prevalent in those with compromised immune systems or those taking certain drugs.

Treatment typically entails the use of antibiotic medications.

A. Indications of tongue disorders: Depending on the specific illness, the symptoms can exhibit significant variation, although they may encompass:

i. Tongue soreness or discomfort.
ii. Edema (Swelling) or hypertrophy.
iii. Variations in colour (white, yellow, black, or red).
iv. The tongue's mobility is limited.
v. Distorted gustatory perceptions.
vi. The tongue may develop lesions or fractures on its surface.

Factors contributing to tongue disorders: Numerous factors, such as the following, can cause tongue diseases:

a. Infections caused by bacteria, viruses, or fungi can result in inflammation and other symptoms.
b. Nutritional deficiencies, namely the absence of vital vitamins and minerals, can impact the health of the tongue.
c. Trauma: Tongue injury from bites or burns can cause inflammation and discomfort.
d. Medical Conditions: Tongue symptoms might be indicative of systemic illnesses such as diabetes, autoimmune disorders, and some cancers.

Therapy and Prophylaxis: The treatment of tongue issues often relies on the root cause of the condition, some general suggestions include practicing proper dental hygiene by regularly brushing, flossing, and utilizing a tongue scraper.

It is important to minimize or prevent the exposure to irritants such as smoke and certain habitual foods that might worsen symptoms.

Related questions from unit 4

1. Draw a neat diagram of neuron and compare between myelinated and non-myelinated neuron.
2. Summarize the action potential process.
3. Evaluate the structure and functions of the sympathetic nervous system.
4. Evaluate the structure and functions of parasympathetic nervous system.
5. Evaluate the structure and functions of eye and ear.
6. Evaluate the structure and function of nose and tongue.
7. Explain the structure and function of the sympathetic nervous system.
8. Explain spinal nerve.
9. Explain the structure and function of a human eye.
10. Explain the structure and function of a human ear.
11. Explain the structure and function of nose.
12. Explain in detail about the disorders of special senses.
13. Explain cranial nerves.
14. Explain in detail about the human tongue

Unit – 5.

Topic	Page no.
Chapter 1: Cardiovascular system	**134 – 136**
1.1. Heart – anatomy of heart	136 – 138
1.2. Blood circulation	138
1.3. Blood vessels	138 – 141
1.4. Structure and functions of artery	141 – 142
1.5. Structure and functions of vein	142 – 144
1.6. Structure and functions of capillaries	144 – 146
1.7. Elements of conduction system of heart	146 – 147
1.8. Heart beat	147 – 148
1.9. Cardiac output	148 – 150
1.10. Cardiac cycle	150 – 152
1.11. Regulation of blood pressure	152 – 153
1.12. Pulse	153 – 155
1.13. Electrocardiogram	155 – 156

1.14. Disorders of heart	156 – 157

Related questions from unit 5	158

Unit – 5.

Chapter 1.

Cardiovascular system.

The cardiovascular system, mostly referred to as the circulatory system, is an essential organ system that carries out the function to carry blood, nutrients, oxygen, carbon dioxide, and waste products throughout the whole body. The heart, blood vessels (such as arteries, veins, and capillaries), and blood essentially make up the cardiovascular system.

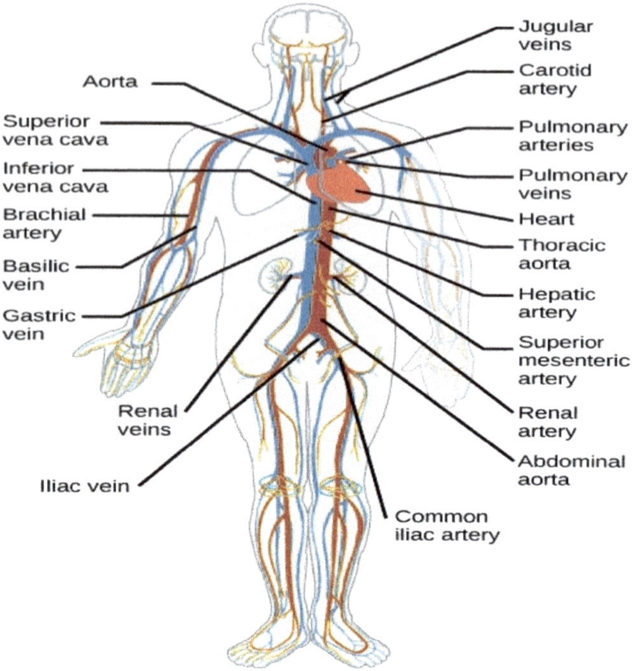

Fig. 59. Cardiovascular system.

Constituents of the cardiovascular system:

a. The heart: The heart is a muscular (contractile) organ that serves as a pump for circulating blood. It possesses a total of four compartments: i.e. Right atrium, left atrium, right ventricles and left ventricles.

i. The atria or atrium, which are the upper chambers of the heart, have specific functions, the right atrium gets blood that lacks oxygen from the body, while the left atrium receives fluid that is rich in oxygen from the lungs.

ii. The ventricles, which are the bottom chambers of the heart, have specific functions; the right ventricle is responsible for pumping deoxygenated blood to the lungs in order to get oxygen, while the left ventricle pumps oxygenated blood throughout the rest of the body.

The heart functions by undergoing a sequence of contraction (systole) and relaxation (diastole), while valves guarantee the passage of blood in one direction between the chambers and out to the arteries.

Cardiovascular system:

The classification of blood vessels is based on three primary types:
a. Arteries transport oxygenated blood from the heart to the body's tissues.
b. Veins transport deoxygenated blood back to the heart.
c. Capillaries are tiny blood veins that allow gases, nutrients, and waste to exchange between the blood and tissues.

A. Circulatory pathways: The cardiovascular system consists of two main circuits:
a. The systemic circulation is responsible for transporting oxygenated blood from the left side of the heart to the body and returning deoxygenated blood to the right side of the heart.
b. The pulmonary circulation is responsible for carrying deoxygenated blood from the right side of the heart to the lungs, where it undergoes gas exchange, this process releases carbon dioxide and receives oxygen, the left side of the heart then receives the oxygenated blood.

Functions: The cardiovascular system performs several functions throughout the body, those are:
i. Blood facilitates the transportation of vital nutrients and oxygen to cells throughout the body.
ii. Waste Removal: The system collects waste products from cells, such as carbon dioxide, and transports them to excretory organs.
iii. Body temperature regulation is a critical process that ensures homeostasis by controlling both blood flow and temperature.
iv. Enhancing immune function: The circulatory system carries immune cells that aid in protecting the body against harmful microorganisms.

Common cardiovascular disorders: The cardiovascular system can be impacted by various factors, including:
a. Coronary artery disease refers to the constriction of the blood vessels that provide oxygenated blood to the heart muscle, which frequently results in heart attacks.
b. Heart failure is a medical disorder characterized by the heart's inability to adequately pump blood to fulfil the body's requirements.
c. Arrhythmias are irregular heart rhythms that can result in a range of problems.
d. Hypertension refers to elevated blood pressure levels, which significantly raise the chances of developing heart disease and stroke.

1.1. Heart: Anatomy of heart:

The heart is a vital organ responsible for pumping blood throughout the body, the atrium, ventricles, valves, and blood vessels comprise its composition. The heart is an intricate cardiac organ vital for circulating blood throughout the body. It is located in the thoracic cavity, between the lungs, and slightly to the left of the sternum.

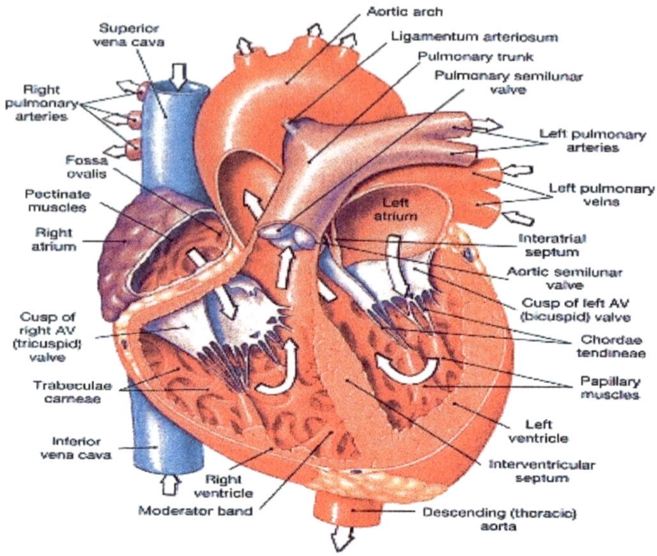

Fig. 60. Anatomy of heart.

The key characteristics are:

i. Size and shape: The heart has approximate dimensions of 12 cm in length, 8.5 cm in breadth, and 6 cm in thickness, making it comparable in size to a closed fist of an individual, the weight of male's heart is roughly 310 grams, while females' heart are around 255 grams.

ii. Location: It is in the central part of the mediastinum, positioned behind the sternum, approximately one-third of its mass is on the right side, while two-thirds are on the left side.

Cardiac chambers: There are four chambers in the heart, divided into two halves:

a. The atria (superior or upper chambers):

i. The right atrium receives unoxygenated blood from the body through the superior and inferior venacava.

ii. The left atrium receives oxygenated blood from the lungs via the pulmonary veins.

b. Ventricles (inferior or lower chambers):

i. The right ventricle propels unoxygenated blood to the lungs through the pulmonary artery.ii. The left ventricle is responsible for propelling oxygenated blood throughout the body via the aorta.

Septa: The heart is partitioned by septa:
a. The interatrial septum is a structure that divides the right and left atria.
b. The interventricular septum is a structure that divides the right and left ventricles.

Cardiac valves: The heart has four primary valves that guarantee the flow of blood in a single direction:
a. Atrioventricular valves:
i. The tricuspid valve is located between the right atrium and right ventricle.
ii. The mitral (bicuspid) valve is located between the left atrium and left ventricle.
b. Semilunar valves: The pulmonary valve is located between the right ventricle and the pulmonary artery.
The aortic valve is located between the left ventricle and the aorta.

Anatomy of the heart wall: The heart wall consists of three layers:
a. The epicardium is part of the pericardium, the outer layer of the heart, its purpose is to provide protection and lubrication.
b. The myocardium is the dense and muscular main layer of the heart that is responsible for its pumping activity. It possesses specific muscle fibers that enable contraction.
c. The endocardium is the innermost layer that lines the heart chambers and covers the valves to prevent blood from adhering and forming clots.

1.2. Blood Circulation:

The heart gets blood via the coronary arteries, which originate from the aorta, the role of these arteries is to deliver oxygenated blood to the cardiac muscle, thus maintaining its optimal functioning, blood circulation refers to the uninterrupted flow of blood throughout the body, propelled by the rhythmic contractions of the heart, the process of pumping oxygenated blood from the heart to the rest of the body, delivering oxygen and nutrients to the tissues and organs, is known as systemic circulation.

The left ventricle propels oxygenated blood into the aorta, arteries transport blood to smaller arterioles and capillaries, where tissues receive oxygen and nutrients. Venules and veins collect deoxygenated blood and transport it back to the right atrium of the heart.

Blood circulates through the lungs, particularly through the pulmonary arteries and veins, the right ventricle propels unoxygenated blood into the pulmonary artery, the lungs receive the blood, expel carbon dioxide, and assimilate oxygen, the pulmonary veins transport oxygenated blood back to the left atrium of the heart.

The role of the heart:

a. The heart functions as a dual pump, where the right side propels deoxygenated blood to the lungs and the left side propels oxygenated blood to the body.

b. The heart's four chambers and valves guarantee unidirectional blood circulation.

c. Arteries transport blood away from the heart, whereas veins bring it back, capillaries are the tiniest blood vessels in which gas and nutrients exchange between the blood and tissues.

d. The circulatory system is vital for the transportation of oxygen, nutrients, hormones, and immune cells to tissues while simultaneously eliminating waste products such as carbon dioxide, it ensuring the proper functioning of the cardiovascular system is essential for overall health and wellness.

1.3. Blood vessels:

Blood veins are vital constituents of the circulatory system, with the primary function of conveying blood throughout the body, we can categorize these into three primary types: arteries, veins, and capillaries, each of which fulfils specific roles and possesses distinctive anatomical features.

Blood vessel classification:

I. Arteries: Arteries transport blood in a direction away from the heart, typically, these structures consist of thick walls and exhibit elasticity, which allows them to withstand and regulate the high blood pressure that the heart expels.

Arteries are composed of three layers:

i. A layer of endothelial cells makes up the tunica intima, which is the innermost layer.

ii. The tunica media is the middle layer of a blood vessel, consisting mostly of smooth muscle and elastic tissue. This layer enables the blood vessel to expand (vasodilation) or contract (vasoconstriction).

iii. The outside layer of connective tissue, known as the tunica externa or adventitia, provides structural support.

Arterial classifications:
i. Elastic arteries, such as the aorta, are large blood vessels that have the ability to stretch and contract in order to accommodate the flow of blood.
ii. Muscular arteries are a type of medium-sized artery that are responsible for distributing blood to certain parts of the body.
iii. Arterioles are the tiniest arteries that control the flow of blood into capillary beds.

II. Capillaries: Capillaries are the tiniest and most abundant blood vessels that link the arterial and venous systems. They enable the transfer of oxygen, nutrients, and waste substances between the bloodstream and body tissues. Capillaries possess a structure characterized by extremely thin walls composed of a solitary layer of endothelial cells, facilitating the effortless transport of molecules.

Function: Capillaries provide widespread tissue vascularization, promoting efficient substance exchange. Their density varies depending on the tissue's metabolic activity. Muscles and organs such as the liver and kidneys have abundant capillary networks, whereas others, such as the cornea, do not have capillaries.

III. Veins: Veins transport blood towards the heart and possess walls that are thinner compared to arteries, owing to the reduced pressure within veins.

Veins, similar to arteries, consist of three layers:
a. The valves in the tunica intima function to prevent blood from flowing backward.
b. The tunica media in veins is thinner compared to arteries and has a lower amount of smooth muscle.
c. The tunica externa is thicker in veins than arteries because it provides structural support.

Vein classifications:
i. Venules are tiny veins that gather blood from capillaries.
ii. Medium and large Veins: These veins transport blood back to the heart; the superior and inferior venacava are the largest veins, carrying deoxygenated blood from the body to the right atrium.

Pathway of blood circulation:

i. Oxygenated Blood: The left ventricle pumps blood into the aorta, which then distributes oxygen-rich blood through systemic arteries to tissues.
In capillary beds, oxygen and nutrients are exchanged for carbon dioxide and waste materials.
ii. Deoxygenated Blood: Venules, veins, and the superior and inferior venacava transport the blood back to the right atrium. The pulmonary arteries carry the right ventricle's deoxygenated blood to the lungs for oxygenation. The pulmonary veins then return the oxygenated blood to the left atrium.

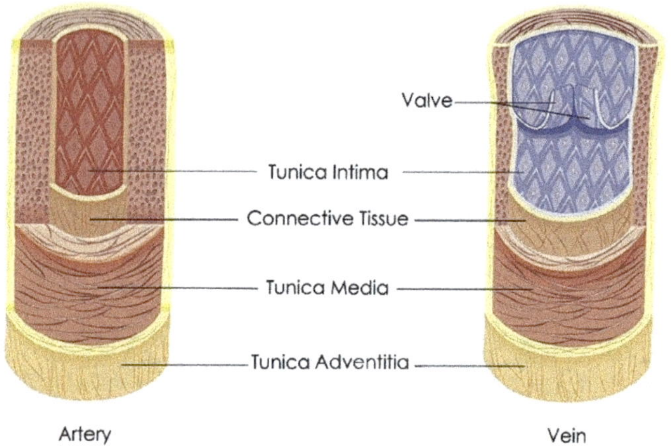

Fig. 61. Anatomy of arteries and veins.

1.4. Structure and functions of artery:
Arteries are crucial blood veins responsible for carrying oxygenated blood from the heart to different tissues and organs in the body. They possess a distinct configuration that allows them to withstand the elevated pressure generated by the heart's pumping mechanism.

Anatomy of Arteries:
Arteries consist of three separate layers, referred to as tunics:
a. The tunica intima is the innermost layer of a blood vessel, a sleek endothelial lining makes up the innermost layer of the artery, reducing friction during blood passage, additionally, it has a thin layer of connective tissue and elastic fibers.

Purpose: This layer facilitates blood flow by creating a frictionless surface and helps prevent clot formation.

b. The tunica media:
The intermediate layer consists mostly of smooth muscle and elastic fibers. The tunica media is more substantial in bigger arteries, such as the aorta, and enables substantial flexibility and contractility.
Purpose: The tunica media plays a vital role in the regulation of blood pressure and blood flow. The blood vessels have the ability to undergo vasoconstriction or vasodilation in response to different stimuli, which helps to regulate blood pressure and ensure efficient blood distribution throughout the body.

c. The tunica externa, also known as the adventitia, is the outermost layer of a blood vessel, the outermost layer consists mostly of collagen fibers, which serve to give structural support and elasticity, connective tissue makes up this layer.

This layer's function is to secure the artery to the surrounding tissues and house larger blood vessels (vasa vasorum) that provide blood flow to the artery itself.

Arterial Classifications:
Classification of arteries based on their anatomical and physiological characteristics:
i. Elastic arteries: Aorta and pulmonary arteries are illustrated.
Characteristics: These arteries include a significant amount of elastic fibers in their walls, enabling them to expand and contract in response to each pulse. This flexibility helps to maintain blood pressure during diastole, which is the heart's relaxation phase.
ii. Muscular arteries: Examples of arteries include the brachial artery and the femoral artery.
Features: These arteries have an increased tunica medium thickness, a greater amount of smooth muscle, and a reduced number of elastic fibers.
Their main role is to distribute blood to particular parts of the body, and they have the ability to control blood flow by constricting or dilating blood vessels.

iii. Arterioles: These are small blood vessels that branch out from arteries.
Definition: Arterioles are the tiniest blood vessels that connect larger arteries to capillaries.

Arterioles have a crucial function in controlling the flow of blood into capillary beds and are important locations for regulating blood pressure.

Functions:
Arteries serve a variety of functions in the body:
a. Oxygenated blood transport:
i. Arteries transport oxygenated blood from the heart to the body's tissues, providing vital nutrients and oxygen required for cellular metabolism.

ii. The second step is the control of blood pressure, arteries are able to regulate blood pressure by adjusting their diameter, coordinating to the presence of smooth muscle in the tunica media, vasoconstriction leads to an elevation in resistance and blood pressure, whereas vasodilation results in a reduction in resistance and blood pressure.

iii. The third step is the regulation of the circulatory system, arteries possess elasticity, which allows them to expand and accommodate the increased volume of blood pumped by the heart during sleep, this elasticity also permits the arteries to sustain a continuous flow of blood during diastole, this elasticity property aids in reducing the pressure fluctuations caused by the heart's pulsations.

iv. Blood distribution: Arteries are divided into smaller arteries, ensuring an equitable distribution of blood to all tissues and organs, thereby facilitating their metabolic requirements.

1.5. Structure and functions of veins:
Veins are a kind of blood vessel responsible for transporting deoxygenated blood from the body's tissues back to the heart. They possess a distinctive anatomical arrangement that enables them to effectively convey blood at a reduced pressure.

Anatomy of Veins:
Veins consist of three different layers, which are comparable to those seen in arteries:
a. The tunica intima is the innermost layer of a blood vessel, a sleek endothelial lining that reduces friction during blood passage makes up the innermost layer of the vein. Additionally, it has a thin stratum of connective tissue.
Purpose: This layer facilitates unobstructed blood flow and helps to prevent clot formation.

b. The tunica media is the intermediate layer consists mostly of connective tissue with elastic fibers and a minor number of smooth muscle cells. This layer's thickness is less than that of arteries, the primary function of the tunica media is to control the diameter of veins and enhance their flexibility.

c. The tunica externa, also known as the adventitia, is the outermost layer of a blood vessel, the outermost layer consists of connective tissue, predominantly composed of collagen fibers, which offers both structural support and elasticity.

This layer serves two purposes: To secure the vein to the surrounding tissues and to house small blood vessels (vasa vasorum) that provide nourishment to the vein.

Categories of veins: We can categorize veins based on their anatomical position and the specific type of blood they transport.
I. Subcutaneous veins: Because they are so close to the body's surface, superficial veins are commonly visible through the skin, examples of veins include the cephalic vein and the basilic vein.
II. Deep veins: Deeply positioned blood vessels commonly observed alongside arteries, the femoral vein and the brachial vein are two examples.
III. Pulmonary veins: Veins that carry oxygenated blood from the lungs to the left atrium of the heart are described.
IV. Systemic veins: Veins that collect deoxygenated blood from the body's tissues and transport it to the right atrium of the heart, examples: superior vena cava, inferior vena cava.

Functions of veins:
1. Blood transportation: Veins collect deoxygenated blood from the body's tissues and return it to the heart for reoxygenation and recirculation.
2. Blood reservoir: Veins can store a significant amount of blood, acting as blood reservoirs. They have a high capacitance, meaning they can expand to accommodate a large volume of blood at low pressure.
3. Venous return: Several factors, including the pumping action of skeletal muscle contractions, the negative pressure in the thorax during inhalation, and the presence of venous valves, contribute to the low pressure in veins.
4. Blood flow regulation: Veins can constrict or dilate in response to various stimuli, helping regulate blood flow and distribution.

Venous valves:

i. One-way venous valves, particularly in the limbs, equip veins to prevent blood backflow, these valves are crucial for maintaining the unidirectional flow of blood towards the heart, particularly against the pull of gravity.

1.6. Structure and functions of capillaries: Capillaries are the smallest and most numerous blood vessels in the circulatory system, playing a crucial role in the exchange of substances between the blood and surrounding tissues.

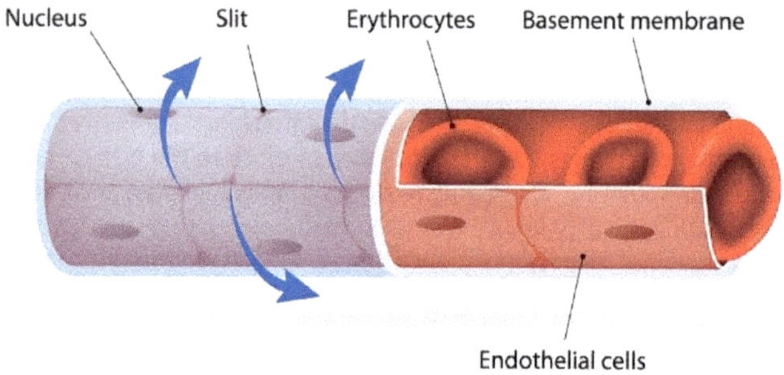

Fig. 62. Anatomy of capillaries.

Structure of Capillaries:
General Features:
Diameter: Capillaries typically measure about 5 to 10 micro-meters in diameter, allowing red blood cells to pass through in a single file, capillary walls consist of a single layer of endothelial cells, serving as a thin barrier for substance exchange, a basement membrane surrounds this layer, providing structural support.

Types of capillaries:
There are three main types of capillaries, each with distinct structural features that facilitate their specific functions:
i. Continuous capillaries:
Structure: These capillaries have a continuous endothelial lining with tight junctions between cells, allowing only small molecules (like ions and water) to pass through.
Location: Found in muscle tissue, skin, and the central nervous system (notably forming the blood-brain barrier).

Function: They provide a selective barrier, limiting the movement of larger substances and maintaining a stable environment for brain tissue.

ii. Fenestrated Capillaries:
Structure: These capillaries have small pores (fenestrations) in their endothelial walls, in addition to intercellular clefts.
Location: Commonly found in the kidneys, small intestine, and endocrine glands.
Function: The pores allow for increased permeability, facilitating the rapid exchange of larger molecules and fluids, which is essential for processes like nutrient absorption and filtration.

iii. Sinusoidal Capillaries
Structure: These are the "leakiest" type of capillary, with large gaps and incomplete basement membranes that allow even larger molecules and cells to pass through.
Location: Found in the liver, spleen, and bone marrow.
Function: They facilitate the exchange of large proteins and blood cells, playing a critical role in processes such as blood cell production and red blood cell recycling.

Functions of capillaries:
a. Exchange of substances:
Capillaries are primarily responsible for the exchange of oxygen, nutrients, carbon dioxide, and waste products between blood and tissues.
This exchange occurs through:
i. Passive Diffusion: Substances move from higher concentrations to lower concentrations, such as oxygen moving from blood to tissues. Pinocytosis: Through this process, cells can actively take in small molecules, allowing for the absorption of nutrients and proteins.

ii. Blood flow regulation:
Capillaries form networks known as capillary beds, which connect arterioles (small arteries) to venules (small veins). Precapillary sphincters, smooth muscle bands that can constrict or dilate to control blood flow based on the metabolic needs of the tissues, regulate the flow of blood into these beds.

iii. Immune function:
Capillaries allow white blood cells to exit the bloodstream and enter tissues to respond to infections or inflammation. This is crucial for the body's immune response.

iv. Maintenance of tissue fluid:
Those balanced capillaries play a role in maintaining fluid balance in tissues by exchanging plasma and interstitial fluid. This process is critical for homeostasis and cell function.

1.7. Elements of conduction system of heart:
The conduction system of the heart is a specialized network of cardiac muscle cells that generates and transmits electrical impulses, coordinating the heart's contractions and maintaining an effective heartbeat, here's a detailed overview of the elements of the conduction system and how they contribute to the heartbeat.

Elements of the Conduction System:

a. Sinoatrial Node (SA Node):
Location: Situated on the upper wall of the right atrium, near the entrance to the superior vena cava.
Function: Known as the heart's natural pacemaker, the SA node generates electrical impulses that initiate each heartbeat. It sets the rhythm for the entire heart by triggering atrial contractions.
Regulation: The autonomic nervous system influences the firing rate of the SA node, with the sympathetic nervous system increasing the heart rate and the parasympathetic nervous system decreasing it.

b. Atrioventricular Node (AV Node):
Location: Situated at the junction of the atria and ventricles, specifically in the interatrial septum.
Function: The AV node receives impulses from the SA node and serves as a gatekeeper, delaying the signal by approximately 120 milliseconds. This delay allows the atria to fully contract and empty their blood into the ventricles before ventricular contraction occurs.
Secondary pacemaker: If the SA node fails, the AV node can take over as a secondary pacemaker, but it generates impulses at a slower rate.

c. Bundle of His (Atrioventricular Bundle):
The location extends from the AV node down the interventricular septum.
Function: The His bundle conducts the electrical impulses from the AV node to the ventricles. It splits into right and left bundle branches, which further transmit the impulse to the respective ventricles.

d. Purkinje fibers:

Location: Spread throughout the ventricular walls, branching from the bundle branches.
Function: Purkinje fibers rapidly conduct the electrical impulse to the ventricular myocardium, causing the ventricles to contract almost simultaneously. This ensures efficient blood flow to the lungs and the rest of the body.

1.8. Heart beat:

The heartbeat process is conduction system initiates coordinated electrical activity, which leads to the heartbeat. The following sequence outlines the process:
a. Impulse generation: The SA node generates an electrical impulse that spreads across the atria, causing them to contract (atrial systole).
b. Signal delay: The AV node delays the impulse to give the ventricles time to fill with blood.
c. Impulse transmission: After the delay, the impulse travels down the "bundle of His", splitting into right and left bundle branches.
d. Ventricular contraction: The Purkinje fibers conduct the impulse, which causes the ventricles to contract in unison (ventricular systole), pumping blood into the pulmonary artery and aorta.
e. Repolarization: After contraction, the heart muscle cells repolarize, preparing for the next heartbeat.

The Autonomic nervous system regulates:
The Autonomic Nervous System (ANS) plays a crucial role in regulating various bodily functions by acting on internal organs, smooth muscles, and glands. The sympathetic nervous system and the parasympathetic nervous system are the two main branches that operate largely unconsciously. These two systems work together to maintain homeostasis and respond to different situations.

The Sympathetic nervous system regulates:
Human often refer to the sympathetic nervous system as the "fight-or-flight" system. The sympathetic nervous system prepares the body for stressful or emergency situations by the heart's rate and the force of its contractions are increasing, dilating the airways to make breathing easier.

Releasing stored energy and increasing muscular strength causing palms to sweat, pupils to dilate, and hair to stand on end slowing down less important processes like digestion and urination.

Regulation by the Parasympathetic nervous system:

The parasympathetic nervous system is known as the "rest and digest" or "feed and breed" system. It controls body processes during ordinary situations and generally conserves and restores. It slows the heart rate and decreases blood pressure.

It stimulates the digestive tract to process food and eliminate waste. This increases digestive secretions and reduces the heartbeat. It constricts the pupils and contracts the ciliary muscles, facilitating closer vision. stimulates sexual arousal and orgasm.

The Autonomic Nervous System's Neurotransmitters:
The two main chemical messengers (neurotransmitters) used for communication within the autonomic nervous system are:
a. Acetylcholine generally has parasympathetic effects.
b. Norepinephrine generally has sympathetic effects.

Regulation by the Enteric Nervous System:
The enteric nervous system is sometimes considered a part of the autonomic nervous system. It contains more than 100 million neurons and controls the gastrointestinal tract. It can work independently or in response to communications from the sympathetic and parasympathetic systems.

1.9. Cardiac output:
Cardiac output (CO) is a critical physiological measurement that represents the volume of blood pumped by the heart per minute. It is essential for ensuring that all body tissues receive adequate oxygen and nutrients to function properly. Here's a detailed overview of cardiac output, including its definition, calculation, factors affecting it, and regulation.

Definition of Cardiac Output: The amount of blood each heart ventricle ejects per minute is called cardiac output. It is a key indicator of cardiovascular health and is crucial for maintaining adequate tissue perfusion.

Formula
The formula for calculating cardiac output is: $CO=HR\times SV$
Where:
CO = cardiac output (in liters per minute).
HR = heart rate (in beats per minute).
SV = stroke volume (the amount of blood pumped from the left ventricle per beat, typically measured in milliliters).

For a healthy individual at rest, the average cardiac output is approximately 5 liters per minute, which can increase significantly during physical activity to meet the body's metabolic demands.

Factors affecting cardiac output:

Several factors influence cardiac output, primarily through changes in heart rate and stroke volume:

I. Heart Rate (HR)

Definition: The number of times the heart beats per minute. Influence: An increase in heart rate generally leads to an increase in cardiac output, provided that stroke volume remains stable. However, if the heart rate increases too much, it can reduce the time available for the ventricles to fill, potentially decreasing stroke volume and, consequently, cardiac output.

II. Stroke Volume (SV)

Definition: The amount of blood ejected by the left ventricle with each heartbeat.

Influence: Stroke volume is affected by:

a. Preload: The degree of stretch in the heart muscle before contraction, influenced by venous return.

b. Contractility: Sympathetic stimulation and certain hormones can strengthen the heart's contraction.

c. Afterload: The resistance the heart must overcome to eject blood; higher afterload can reduce stroke volume.

III. Venous Return:

Definition: The amount of blood returning to the heart from the body. Influence: increased venous return enhances preload, which can increase stroke volume and, thereby, cardiac output.

IV. The autonomic nervous system:

The sympathetic nervous system increases heart rate and contractility, resulting in increased cardiac output during stress or exercise.

The Parasympathetic Nervous System decreases heart rate, which can reduce cardiac output under resting conditions.

V. Hormonal Regulation:

Hormones such as adrenaline (epinephrine) and norepinephrine increase heart rate and contractility, enhancing cardiac output. Other hormones, such as those involved in fluid balance (e.g., aldosterone, antidiuretic hormone), can affect blood volume and venous return.

VI. Physical Activity:
During exercise, the body's demand for oxygen increases, leading to higher heart rates and stroke volumes, significantly raising cardiac output.

VII. Body position:
Changes in body position (e.g., standing up from a lying position) can affect venous return and, consequently, cardiac output.

Measurement of Cardiac Output:
You can measure cardiac output using a variety of techniques, including
a. Echocardiography: non-invasive imaging to estimate stroke volume and cardiac output.
b. Doppler ultrasound: measures blood flow velocity to estimate cardiac output.
c. Thermodilution is an invasive method commonly used in critical care settings to directly measure cardiac output.

1.10. Cardiac cycle:
The cardiac cycle refers to the sequence of events that occur during one complete heartbeat, encompassing the contraction and relaxation of the heart chambers. It is crucial for maintaining efficient blood flow throughout the body. The cycle consists of two main phases: systole (contraction) and diastole (relaxation). Here's a detailed overview of the cardiac cycle:

Phases of the Cardiac Cycle:
I. Atrial Systole:
Description: This phase begins when the sinoatrial (SA) node generates an electrical impulse, causing the atria to contract.

The open atrioventricular (AV) valves (tricuspid and mitral valves) push blood from the atria into the ventricles.
Duration: This phase lasts approximately 0.1 seconds.

II. Ventricular Systole:
When the atrium systole happens, an electrical impulse goes to the atrioventricular (AV) node and then through the bundle of His and Purkinje fibers, making the ventricles contract.
Function:
The pressure in the ventricles rises, closing the AV valves to prevent backflow into the atria.

The open semilunar valves (pulmonary and aortic valves) eject blood into the pulmonary artery from the right ventricle and the aorta from the left ventricle.
Duration: This phase lasts about 0.3 seconds.

3. Ventricular Diastole:
Description: After ventricular systole, the ventricles relax, and the pressure within them decreases.
Function:
To prevent backflow from the arteries into the ventricles, the semilunar valves are closed.
As the AV valves open, blood flows from the atrium into the ventricles, filling them with blood.
Duration: This phase lasts approximately 0.4 seconds.

4. Atrial Diastole:
Description: While the ventricles are filling, the atria are also in a relaxed state, allowing them to fill with blood returning from the body (via the superior and inferior venacava) and from the lungs (via the pulmonary veins).
Function: This phase prepares the atria for the next cycle of contraction.

Overview of the Cardiac Cycle:
The entire cardiac cycle typically lasts about 0.8 seconds at a resting heart rate of 75 beats per minute, we can summarize the cycle as follows:
i. Atrial Systole: Atria contract, filling ventricles.
ii. Ventricular Systole: The vesicles contract, ejecting blood into the arteries.
iii. Ventricular Diastole: When the atria fills with blood, the vesicles relax.
iv. Atrial Diastole: The atria relaxes and fills with blood.

v. Regulation of the Cardiac Cycle:
The heart's conduction system, primarily the SA node, which acts as the pacemaker, regulates the cardiac cycle. The autonomic nervous system also influences heart rate and contractility.

Sympathetic Nervous System: Increases heart rate and the force of contractions during stress or physical activity.

The Parasympathetic Nervous System is responsible for reducing heart rate and promoting relaxation during rest.

1.11. Regulating blood pressure:

Blood pressure regulation is a complex process that involves multiple mechanisms to maintain adequate blood flow and pressure throughout the body. This regulation is essential for ensuring that tissues receive sufficient oxygen and nutrients while removing waste products. The following is an overview of the key factors and mechanisms involved in blood pressure regulation.

Blood pressure regulation's key mechanisms:

a. Neural regulation:

The autonomic nervous system plays a crucial role in regulating blood pressure through the sympathetic and parasympathetic branches. Sympathetic Nervous System: Activation leads to vasoconstriction (narrowing of blood vessels), increased heart rate, and enhanced heart contractility, all of which raise blood pressure. Norepinephrine is the primary neurotransmitter involved in this response.

The Parasympathetic Nervous System, primarily activated through the vagus nerve, lowers heart rate, which in turn can lower blood pressure. This pathway uses acetylcholine as the neurotransmitter.

b. Hormonal regulation:

Several hormones control blood pressure by affecting blood volume and vascular resistance:

i. Renin-Angiotensin-Aldosterone System (RAAS):

The kidneys release renin in response to low blood pressure or low sodium levels.

ii. Renin transforms angiotensinogen from the liver into angiotensin I, which the lungs' angiotensin-converting enzyme (ACE) then converts to angiotensin II, angiotensin II causes vasoconstriction and stimulates aldosterone release from the adrenal glands, promoting sodium and water retention that increase blood volume and pressure.

iii. Antidiuretic Hormone (ADH): Released from the posterior pituitary gland, ADH promotes water reabsorption in the kidneys, increasing blood volume and pressure.

iv. Natriuretic Peptides: The heart releases hormones such as atrial natriuretic peptide (ANP) in response to increased blood volume and pressure. They promote vasodilation and increase sodium excretion, leading to reduced blood pressure.

c. Local regulation:

Localized regulation of blood flow and pressure within tissues can also occur:

i. Autoregulation: tissues can regulate their own blood flow based on their metabolic needs. For example, during increased activity, muscles require more oxygen, leading to vasodilation of the arterioles supplying those muscles.
ii. Vasodilators and Vasoconstrictors: Local factors such as carbon dioxide levels, pH, and oxygen levels can influence smooth muscle contraction in blood vessels. high carbon dioxide and low pH typically promote vasodilation, while high oxygen levels can lead to vasoconstriction in certain tissues.

d. Baroreceptor Reflex:
Baroreceptors are specialized sensors located in the walls of blood vessels (particularly in the carotid arteries and aorta) that detect blood pressure changes, when blood pressure rises, baroreceptors send signals to the central nervous system, which responds by decreasing heart rate, causing vasodilation, and lowering blood pressure.
Conversely, when blood pressure drops, the baroreceptors signal for an increase in heart rate and vasoconstriction to raise blood pressure.

e. Other factors:
i. Blood Volume: Changes in blood volume directly affect blood pressure. Increased blood volume (due to fluid retention) raises blood pressure, while decreased volume (due to bleeding or dehydration) lowers it.
ii. Physical Activity: During exercise, blood pressure rises due to increased cardiac output and vasoconstriction in non-active tissues, while vasodilation occurs in active muscles.

1.12. Pulse:

The heart pumps blood through the arteries, causing them to expand and contract rhythmically. It serves as a vital indicator of cardiovascular health and can provide insights into heart rate, rhythm, and overall circulatory function.

Definition of Pulse: The heart contraction, specifically during ventricular systole, ejects blood into the arteries, generating a pressure wave that results in the pulse. This pressure wave travels through the arterial system, causing the arteries to expand and then retract.

Characteristics of Pulse:
a. Rate: The pulse rate is the number of beats per minute (bpm), a normal resting pulse rate for adults typically ranges from 60 to 100 bpm, although it can vary based on factors such as age, fitness level, and overall health.

b. Rhythm: The pulse's rhythm refers to the beats' regularity, a regular pulse has consistent intervals between beats, while an irregular pulse may indicate underlying health issues.
c. Strength: The heart can pump a variety of blood volumes, as indicated by the strength of the pulse. A strong pulse suggests excellent blood flow, while a weak or thready pulse may indicate reduced cardiac output or blood volume.
d. Quality: Human can characterize the pulse's quality as bounding, weak, or normal, which reflects the state of the circulatory system.

Locations to Measure Pulse:
Various points on the body, where arteries are close to the surface, can detect the pulse. Common pulse points include:
i. Radial Pulse: Located on the thumb side of the wrist.
ii. Carotid Pulse: Located in the neck, next to the trachea.
iii. The brachial pulse is located in the inner elbow.
iv. The femoral pulse is located in the groin area.
v. The popliteal pulse is located behind the knee.
vi. Dorsalis Pedis Pulse: Found on the top of the foot.
vii. The posterior tibial pulse is located behind the ankle.

Measurement of Pulse: To measure the pulse, follow these steps:
a. Locate the Pulse point: Use your index and middle fingers to gently press over the pulse point (e.g., radial artery at the wrist).
b. Count the Beats: For 30 seconds, count the number of beats and multiply by 2 to get the beats per minute. For more accuracy, especially if the pulse is irregular, count for a full minute.
c. Assess rhythm and strength: Take note of the pulse's rhythm (regular or irregular) and strength (strong, weak, or thready).

Significance of Pulse:
Monitoring the pulse is critical for assessing cardiovascular health. Changes in pulse rate, rhythm, or strength can indicate various health conditions, including: stress, fever, or heart conditions can cause tachycardia, an abnormally high pulse rate.
a. Bradycardia: An abnormally low pulse rate, which can occur during sleep or in well-trained athletes.
b. Arrhythmias: irregular heartbeats that may require medical evaluation.
c. Shock or Hypovolemia: A weak or thready pulse may indicate inadequate blood flow due to shock or significant blood loss.

1.13. Electrocardiogram:

An electrocardiogram (ECG or EKG) is a diagnostic tool that records the electrical activity of the heart over a period of time. It is a widely used test to assess the health of the heart and detect any abnormalities in its rhythm or structure. Here's a concise overview of an electrocardiogram:

Purpose of an ECG:
a. We diagnose heart attacks and other heart conditions.
b. Detect abnormal heart rhythms (arrhythmias).
c. Monitor the effects of certain medications on the heart.
d. Evaluate symptoms such as chest pain, shortness of breath, and palpitations.

How an ECG works?
a. The patient has electrodes applied to their chest, arms, and legs.
b. These electrodes detect the electrical signals generated by the heart and
transmit them to the ECG machine.
c. The machine records these signals and displays them as waveforms on
graph paper or a computer screen.
d. An ECG interpretation: Each wave on the ECG corresponds to a specific event in the heart's electrical cycle.
e. The shape, size, and timing of these waves provide information about the heart's condition.
f. Abnormalities in the waveforms may indicate a variety of heart conditions, including Myocardial infarction (heart attack) Ischemia refers to a decrease in blood flow to the heart, Hypertrophy (enlargement of the heart) Arrhythmias.

Types of ECG:
i. Resting ECG: Performed while the patient is at rest
ii. Stress ECG (Treadmill Test): Performed while the patient is exercising on a treadmill or stationary bike.

iii. Holter Monitor: A portable ECG device worn for 24-48 hours to record the heart's activity over an extended period.
iv. Event Recorder: A portable ECG device used to record the heart's activity when symptoms occur.

Limitations of ECG:

a. ECG may not detect all heart conditions, especially those that occur intermittently.
b. It provides limited information about the heart's structure and function.
c. Additional tests, such as echocardiography or cardiac catheterization, may be necessary for a more comprehensive evaluation.

1.14. Disorders of heart:

Disorders of the heart encompass a wide range of conditions that affect the heart's structure, function, and rhythm. These disorders can lead to significant health complications and may require medical intervention.
Below is an overview of some common heart disorders, their causes, symptoms, and potential treatments.

Common heart disorders:
i. Coronary Artery Disease (CAD):
Description: A condition characterized by the narrowing or blockage of the coronary arteries due to atherosclerosis (buildup of plaque).
Symptoms: chest pain (angina), shortness of breath, fatigue, and heart attacks.
Treatment: Lifestyle changes (diet, exercise), medications (statins, antiplatelet agents), and procedures (angioplasty, coronary artery bypass grafting).

ii. Heart Failure:
Description: A chronic condition where the heart cannot pump blood effectively to meet the body's needs.
Symptoms: fatigue, shortness of breath, fluid retention (swelling in legs and ankles), and rapid heartbeat.
Treatment: medications (diuretics, ACE inhibitors, beta-blockers), lifestyle modifications, and in severe cases, devices like pacemakers or heart transplants.

iii. Arrhythmias:
Abnormal heart rhythms are caused by issues with the heart's electrical system.
Types: atrial fibrillation (AFib), ventricular tachycardia, and bradycardia.
Symptoms: palpitations, dizziness, fainting, or chest discomfort.
Treatment: medications (antiarrhythmics), lifestyle changes, electrical cardioversion, or implantable devices like pacemakers and defibrillators.

iv. Valvular Heart Disease:
Description: Disorders affecting one or more of the heart valves (mitral, aortic, tricuspid, or pulmonary).
Types: stenosis (narrowing of the valve) and regurgitation (leakage of the valve).
Symptoms: fatigue, shortness of breath, palpitations, and swelling in the legs.
Treatment: medications, lifestyle changes, and surgical interventions (valve repair or replacement).

v. Cardiomyopathy:
Description: A group of diseases that affect the heart muscle, leading to decreased heart function.
Types: dilated, hypertrophic, and restrictive cardiomyopathy.
Symptoms: shortness of breath, fatigue, swelling, and irregular heartbeats.
Treatment options include medications, lifestyle changes, and, in severe cases, heart transplants.

vi. Congenital heart defects:
Description: Structural heart problems present at birth, affecting the heart's anatomy and function.
Symptoms: Vary widely; may include cyanosis (bluish skin), rapid breathing, and fatigue.
Treatment: Depends on the defect; may involve medications, catheter procedures, or surgery.

vii. Pericarditis:
Description: Inflammation of the pericardium (the sac surrounding the heart).
Symptoms: sharp chest pain that may worsen with deep breaths or lying down, fever, and fatigue.
Treatment: anti-inflammatory medications, pain relievers, and, in severe cases, procedures to drain excess fluid.

Related questions from unit 5

1. Explain the blood vessels.
2. Summarize the functioning of cardiovascular system with a proper diagram of heart.
3. Describe the structure and function of human heart.
4. Compare and differentiate the about the vein and artery.
5. Explain the blood circulation system in human body.
6. Summarize the cardiac cycle.
7. Describe the structure of human heart.
8. Describe the electrical conduction system of the heart.
9. Describe is the cardiac cycle, and how is it regulated to ensure efficient pumping of blood.
10. Discuss the common cardiovascular diseases.
11. Define congestive heart failure.
12. Describe the term hypertension and pulse rate.
13. Explain following terms: Cardiac output, heart rate, pulse rate, tachycardia, bradycardia, angina pectoris.
14. Explain in brief cardiac output.
15. Describe briefly electrocardiogram.

Rough work page – I

Rough work page 2

www.ingramcontent.com/pod-product-compliance
Ingram Content Group UK Ltd.
Pitfield, Milton Keynes, MK11 3LW, UK
UKHW021400190726
13845UKWH00028B/779